COMMUNITY
HEALTH
NURSING
Evolution and Process

COMMUNITY HEALTH NURSING

Evolution and Process

CATHERINE W. TINKHAM, R.N., B.S., M.P.H.

PROFESSOR AND COORDINATOR
GRADUATE PROGRAM IN COMMUNITY HEALTH NURSING
BOSTON UNIVERSITY SCHOOL OF NURSING
BOSTON, MASSACHUSETTS

ELEANOR F. VOORHIES, B.A., R.N., M.N., M.A.

ASSOCIATE PROFESSOR AND COORDINATOR
COMMUNITY HEALTH NURSING
BOSTON COLLEGE SCHOOL OF NURSING
BOSTON, MASSACHUSETTS

APPLETON-CENTURY-CROFTS
Educational Division
MEREDITH CORPORATION
New York

This book is dedicated to
LULU
with love

C.T. and E.V.

Preface

We are living in exciting times in which the role and responsibilities of all the health professionals are being challenged. The people are demanding comprehensive health care while at the same time professional health workers are becoming more and more specialized, and their problems of communication are increasing. Everyone seems to have discovered the community as the base of operation. This has resulted in an increase in the services which are offered but a decrease in the coordination of these services. New kinds of health workers are appearing almost daily and others are being proposed. Health care is now considered a right to which all people are entitled regardless of their ability to pay.

Amidst all of this chaos, traditional public health and public health nursing programs are undergoing a metamorphosis. The artificial barriers between promotion of health and treatment of disease are disappearing. Emphasis is on the health of the community and how best to meet its health needs. A new partnership is developing in which health professionals from all disciplines and agencies must work together to provide the services demanded by the people. Community health nursing can no longer think of itself as having sole responsibility for nursing outside of the hospital but must work with other specialties within nursing and with other disciplines in order to better serve the people. The old relationships and strict agency prerogatives are no longer relevant. A new role for the community health nurse is evolving. It is imperative that she have the competencies and the vision to meet the challenge and make a contribution with others for improved and more comprehensive health services.

In order to better understand community health nursing today one must look to the past as well as to the present. Nursing, as other professions, did not chart its own course but was molded by the undulating forces of the times. It emerged and organized amidst turbulence and change; developed its own identity in a complex and dynamic society; and became a vital force in its own right. Early in the history of the profession, public health nursing became a specialty because of a need by the people for nursing care of the sick in their own homes. We believe that the overall developments in transportation, immigration and population, industrialization, science and technology, education, social consciousness, the role of government, and the role of women—separate though inexorably related—generated forces which were deciding factors in the evolution of nursing and public health nursing, and are still exerting their influences today. Each of these developments was not equally important simultaneously; however, their interrelatedness was and continues to be omnipresent. Some writers no doubt would select other events and resulting forces and interpret them differently, but we believe those which we have selected were instrumental in bringing about a whole new way of life which made it possible and inescapable for nursing and other professions to be nourished and to grow. Nursing must be increasingly knowledgeable about today's world and recognize and understand the effect of the ebb and flow of societal forces on its practices and responsibilities. It must further develop its own potential as one of the vital forces for a better life.

We have limited our exploration to developments in the United States. This book is divided into three parts—looking to the past, the present, and the future.

Part I includes three chapters. Chapter 1 deals with the period from 1865-1900. We have selected this period following the Civil War as our starting point because it was within this time that the seeds of organized nursing and public health nursing were about ready to burst forth. This was also the period within which the foundations were laid for many of our contemporary health programs and institutions.

Chapter 2 deals with the period from 1900 to the New Deal. It was during this time that organized nursing became viable and standards for education and practice were established. The responsibility of the government for the health of the people became apparent during these years.

Chapter 3 starts with the New Deal and goes through the Johnson era. This period was characterized by explosive developments in science and technology which drastically affected the way of life. Nursing became firmly established as a profession and great strides were made toward education of nurses within institutions of higher learning.

We have focused our attention on some of the changes which occurred in society during these three periods, and which we believe have influenced nursing and public health nursing. We have attempted to show implicitly or explicitly the interrelationships of these changes. What was America like at these times? How did public health nursing evolve as part of public health and as part of nursing? Why did it grow and organize as it did? What were some of the changes in education, in nursing education, and in the status of women which were significant to the development of nursing?

In Part II the major focus is on the process of community health nursing in relation to the family and the community. Forces in society will constantly change and affect the directions in which nursing with other professions will move. It is for this reason that we are emphasizing the process of nursing as we believe the process will remain essentially the same within a changing society.

The term public health nursing has been broadened to community health nursing. This concept refocuses the nurses' concern for the health of the people and puts it where it belongs—in the community itself, thus removing the responsibility from the aegis of specific agencies. It involves the nurse with professional and nonprofessional persons in the community in a broadened and different kind of partnership. What is the relationship of public health nursing organizational patterns to the growing demands of the public for improved health care? What is the influence on community health nursing of the rapidly increasing governmental support of a variety of community health programs? What is the impact on community health nursing of the increased numbers of health workers who have recently discovered the community? What effect has the knowledge explosion had upon community health nursing? What is the relationship between traditional public health nursing services and the needs of a changing, mobile population?

In Part III, we have looked at the road ahead. We have identified some of the assets and liabilities with which community health nursing faces the future; have discussed its developing role as the family health nurse practitioner, and pointed out some of the challenges and pitfalls which undoubtedly lie ahead. Finally, we have indicated some of the implications for nursing education and research.

This book is planned for the use of nursing students in colleges and universities, and for community health nurse practitioners, as well as other community health workers.

We wish to express our thanks and appreciation to Marie Farrell, Dean Emeritus of the Boston University School of Nursing for her perceptiveness, constructive criticism, and support; to our students who unknowingly have contributed many ideas; to Gertrude Smith whose careful and meticulous work contributed immeasurably to the preparation of this manuscript; and finally, to each other, without whom this book would never have been written.

Contents

Preface   vii

PART I   Social Forces Affecting the Development of Nursing and Community Health Nursing   1

CHAPTER 1   The Period From 1865 to 1900   3

CHAPTER 2   The Period From 1900 to the New Deal   29

CHAPTER 3   The Period From the New Deal Through the Johnson Era   62

PART II   Community Health Nursing Process   103

CHAPTER 4   The Scene at the Beginning of the 1970s   105

CHAPTER 5   The Family as the Patient   117

CHAPTER 6   Family Data Collection   130

CHAPTER 7   Analysis of Data and Identification of Family Nursing Needs   146

CHAPTER 8   Developing the Family Nursing Care Plan   159

CHAPTER 9   Implementing and Evaluating the Family Nursing Care Plan   176

CHAPTER 10   The Community as the Patient   193

CHAPTER 11   Gathering Pertinent Data About the Community   205

CHAPTER 12   Analysis of Data and Identification of Community Nursing Needs   220

CHAPTER 13   Developing a Nursing Plan of Action for the Community   236

CHAPTER 14   Implementing and Evaluating a Nursing Plan of Action for the Community   251

PART III   Implications for the Future   267

CHAPTER 15 The Road Ahead   269
Appendix A Family Data Collection   279
Appendix B Community Nursing Survey Guide   287
Index   307

PART I

SOCIAL FORCES AFFECTING THE DEVELOPMENT OF NURSING AND COMMUNITY HEALTH NURSING

CHAPTER 1
The Period
From 1865 to 1900

**The Scene at the Close
of the Civil War**

We will start our exploration of the past by attempting to recapture some of the feelings and aspirations of the American people at the close of the Civil War. We recognize the limitations of this approach, as each person looking back over history will interpret events differently depending upon his background and frame of reference. We will explore the environment in which the people lived: their growing cities; the teeming slums; the deplorable health conditions; the expanding transportation; and the burgeoning industry. We will identify some of the forces and changes which were shaping their way of life; the aftermath of the antislavery agitation; the changing role of women; and the strivings for education.

Although America after the war was primarily rural, cities were developing rapidly and bringing with them problems of housing, sanitation, and health. The population, 31,443,321 in 1860,[1] was growing due to the influence of immigrants from northern and western Europe. Many of these newcomers settled in the crowded slums of the growing cities. This was still a horse-and-buggy era, and goods, passengers, mail, and all manner of things were transported across the country by stagecoach and Pony Express. Railroads were expanding, but they did not link the East with the West. The frontiers of the West were still being settled. The slavocracy of the agrarian South was dissolved and no longer a threat to the entire economy. Industry which, especially in the North, had geared itself to the war effort was now ready to expand.

For a democracy to work there is a need for educated people; this was becoming more and more apparent although only a few states had compulsory school attendance laws. The public school system was in its formative stages, and only a minority of the young people attended high school. In the large eastern cities boys and girls were educated separately. Outside the cities and in the West, where the population was sparse, they were educated together. By the close of the war women had become accepted as the teachers of both boys and girls. Nowhere else in the world had this happened, and it was to have a profound effect on the development of college education for women. Higher education was predominately for men in private colleges which offered classical curricula with strong emphasis on theology. In 1862 Congress had passed the Morrill Act to make possible the establishment in each state of at least one college particularly adapted to the needs of agriculture and industry. The implications of this legislation had not yet become evident.

Women's place was in the home for the rearing and nurturing of children. The superiority of the male was stressed over and over again. Wives and children, along with other chattels, were the property of the husband. In most states married women could neither own property separately from their husbands nor decide about the disposition of property at their death. Women were not allowed to vote. Very few occupations were open to them. Pay for those who were employed was lower than that of men. Prior to the Civil War a few women, both individually and in groups, had actively participated in the rebellion against the system of slavery. They had become involved in public debates and lectures, and some had expressed their

[1] Bureau of the Census. *A Century of Population Growth: 1790-1900*. Washington, D. C., Government Printing Office, 1909, p. 55.

opinions in writing. Harriet Beecher Stowe's *Uncle Tom's Cabin* was widely read and had far-reaching effects. Some of the women in the South had freed their slaves and gone north to campaign against slavery. Paralleling this whole involvement of women in abolition was the beginning of the feminist movement which was to gain momentum after the war and finally result in women's suffrage.

The winds of change affecting the status of women, which had begun prior to the Civil War, were intensified by the war itself. Women had become involved in all aspects of the war effort and had taken over many of the jobs previously held by men. Their accomplishments had equalled and often exceeded those of men. It was largely through the efforts of the women in the North that the Secretary of War, in 1861, approved a document that gave the President the power to appoint a United States Sanitary Commission to oversee the health and welfare of the army and to be a channel of communication between the people and the government.[2] The United States Sanitary Commission became the forerunner of the American Red Cross. Ladies Aid Societies were established in the northern states and were affiliated with the Commission. The women in the Aid Societies had involved themselves with the care of the sick and wounded soldiers, with the provision of supplies for the soldiers on the fighting front, and with the maintenance of contact between the soldiers and the home front. The contribution of these women is graphically described by Greenbie:

> One thing that universally impressed the many gentlemen whose time or money the Ladies' Aid societies commandeered was the "perfect attitude of women for business." By the end of the Civil War, this Sanitary Commission enterprise which the ladies had started, and of which they remained to the end the backbone, was worth about $50,000,000. And in those days that was a very large business enterprise, indeed. They had the cooperation of all railroads and express companies in transporting their stores free, and of the telegraph companies in sending their messages free. They had many and intricate arrangements for cooperation with the army. They had, in all, about 32,000 groups of women, large and small, organized as cooperating Ladies' Aid societies.
>
> To keep this vast network of business in any kind of order was a test of efficiency in detail and in overall organization to which the housewives of the land had risen nobly. As Dr. Bellows said in a message quoted, with endorsement by Limus P. Brockett, a merchant of New York, "A generous emulation among the branches of the United States Sanitary Commission, managed generally by women, usually, however,

[2] Greenbie, M. B. *Lincoln's Daughters of Mercy.* New York, G. P. Putnam's Sons, 1944, pp. 76-77.

with some aid from men, brought their business habits and methods to an almost perfect finish. . . . They acknowledged and answered, endorsed and filed their letters; they sorted their stores and kept an accurate account of stock; they had their books and reports kept in the most approved forms; they balanced their cash accounts with the most painstaking precision; they exacted of each other regularity of attendance and punctiliousness of official etiquette." They did even more than this. They created and introduced into the government records the first complete clerical system any army had ever had. It was their careful registering of the soldiers that formed the basis of the pension system for Civil War veterans.[3]

The women who had been so totally involved in the war effort had found this a rewarding and satisfying experience. They had become less provincial and more nationalistic in their outlook and were loath to return to their former subordinate existence.

Many women and an increasing number of men were beginning to demand opportunities in higher education for women. Matthew Vassar had been tremendously impressed by the ability of women during the war. In 1865 he established Vassar College which was the first college to provide education for women similar to that offered to men in men's colleges.

Health conditions were poor throughout the country, particularly in the crowded slums of the growing cities. The people were continuously plagued by illnesses of all kinds which they accepted as the way of life. Life expectancy at birth was about 41 years.[4] Tuberculosis was endemic and the leading cause of death. Epidemics of cholera, yellow fever, and scarlet fever were still sweeping the country, but were on the wane. The causes of disease were unknown and thought to be due to the environment. Thus, there was great emphasis on sanitation. Medical research was practically nonexistent even in the best medical centers. A few boards of health had been established in some of the cities, but there were no organized public health programs as we know them today.

Hospitals were considered pest houses and looked upon as places in which to die. Their patients were usually the poor and homeless. Nursing care was given by untrained, unqualified men and women who were predominantly from the poorer classes. They had servant or domestic status and were often recruited from the ranks of

---

[3] *Ibid.*, p. 216.
[4] Smillie, W. G. *Public Health—Its Promise for the Future.* New York, The Macmillan Company, 1955, Frontispiece.

prisoners, scrubwomen, and convalescent patients. The majority of the sick were given care at home by female family members or neighbors, many of whom had a great deal of experience in caring for the sick and were respected members of their communities. Organized nursing had not as yet been established, but the influence of Florence Nightingale on the development of trained nurses in England was beginning to be felt in the United States.

There were stirrings of a social consciousness which was expressing itself in various ways and was to become full blown by the end of the century. Many of the women who had had experience as volunteer nurses in the army were anxious to use their knowledge in caring for the people at home. Literature, both fiction and nonfiction, was describing some of the contemporary social problems and making the people more aware of and concerned about the plight of the poor, the conditions of the slums, and the general poor health and sanitary conditions. Compassion for humanity, so sharply expressed through the abolitionist movement, was growing.

The federal government was fairly weak at this time and maintained a "hands off" policy except for some of the overall responsibilities that were specifically stated in the Constitution. Each state assumed major responsibility for its own affairs with little or no relationship to those of other states.

1865 to 1900

The period from the close of the Civil War to the turn of the century was particularly significant in the history of the United States. It was a time of change and turmoil—no less dynamic than that with which we struggle today. It saw what had been a restless, bitterly divided country pick itself up, bind up its wounds, and go forward with hope and optimism for the future.

The Civil War with all its horror and devastation, instead of dividing the country, proved to be a unifying force. Although the wounds were deep and bitter (and some would influence the people for generations) there was a national cohesiveness and sense of unity that had not been apparent before. The rapid expansions on all fronts that occurred between 1865 and 1900 had their beginnings before the war, but it was almost as if the war had unleashed the energies of the people and made it possible for them to move forward as a nation.

Transportation   Some historians say that prog-
                                            ress in transportation was the
                                            most important development
                                            during this period. In 1869 the
completion of the transcontinental railroad linked the East and West
for the first time. The results were profound and far reaching. Great
growth and settlement of the West was made possible, and by the
end of the century the era of the frontiers was over. A more common
culture began to develop. A letter mailed in New York, which
formerly had taken weeks and even months by stage coach, or by the
perilous voyage around the Isthmus of Panama, now reached the
West Coast in a matter of days. Magazines, newspapers, and books
were more readily available. Women in the West learned about
fashions in the East, and the demand for dress patterns and materials
grew. Housewives wanted to purchase new foods and household
goods which were appearing in increasing numbers. A vast new
market clamored for more and diverse machinery and equipment.

Towns sprang up almost overnight along the railroad routes and
became centers for storage and transfer of produce from the large
and small farms and factories throughout the land. Men sweated in
great mills in Pittsburgh and other growing cities, and strained to produce coal and steel for the growing miles of railroad tracks and passenger and freight cars. Americans who previously had been isolated
on small and large farms, particularly in the Middle and Far West, began to travel. Many sought work in and around the cities which were
teeming with businesses and opportunities. By 1900 there were
193,000 miles of railroad.[5] The building of the railroads was primarily a private enterprise. The situation was ripe for businessmen alert
to rich opportunity. They were not found wanting. As the transcontinental lines developed, vast fortunes were made, large companies
were formed, and later great mergers took place. The federal and
state governments gave generous grants of land and financial loans to
the railroad companies. This assistance, however, was often exploited
by the states, many of whom passed legislation geared to their own
interests and unrelated to and at times detrimental to those of other
states. Because of these practices, which were of national concern,
Congress passed the Interstate Commerce Act in 1887, which out-
lawed many of the discriminatory acts of the railroads. This was the
first regulatory legislation passed by the federal government in the

[5] Handlin, O. *The Americans.* Boston, Little, Brown and Company, 1963, p. 270.

interests of society as a whole. Some say it heralded the beginning of the end of individualism in the United States.

The horse and buggy and, in the latter part of the century, the bicycle were the most common modes of transportation, in spite of the growth of the railroads. By 1900 the discovery of electricity had led to the development of trolley cars in the larger cities, and the first subway had been introduced in Boston. A few horseless carriages were appearing in the cities, but there was not much confidence in their future. Dulles quotes a writer of the times:

> "The ordinary 'horseless carriage'," it was pontifically stated by one editorial writer of the day, "is at present a luxury for the wealthy, and although its price will probably fall in the future, it will never, of course, come into common use."[6]

Industrialization

Even though some say that developments in transportation were the most important at this time, the remarkable growth in transportation could not have occurred without the industrial know-how which accompanied it. Scientific and technologic advances made possible new products, equipment, and methods of production. The practical ingenuity of people in America, that is, the ability to apply the fruits of scientific discoveries, both from Europe and the United States, was one of their greatest assets. The discovery of electricity, the incandescent lamp, the telephone, the typewriter, and many other conveniences effected vast changes throughout the nation. Markets grew, not only in America, but in other countries as well. Industrial expansion was favored by rich, untapped natural resources, a ready labor force, investment of capital from abroad, absence of trade barriers, lack of hampering traditions, and the "hands off" policy of the federal government.

The industrial revolution, though primarily a phenomenon of cities, affected every corner of the country. It made possible the mechanization of farming and changed it from an individual occupation to a business venture. Between 1850 and 1900 the number of farm workers doubled; while the value of produce increased twentyfold.[7]

[6]Dulles, F. R. *The United States Since 1865*. Ann Arbor, The University of Michigan Press, 1959, p. 91.
[7]Calhoun, A. W. *A Social History of the American Family*, Vol. III. Cleveland, The Arthur E. Clark Company, 1919, p. 66.

Immigration and Population   Industrialization could not have occurred without a ready supply of labor to meet the demands of industry and farm-ing. In addition to the sons and daughters of farmers and business-men, an endless flow of immigrants supplied the bulk of the migra-tory labor force of agriculture, lumber camps, and construction. Thousands upon thousands of workers poured into the cities to meet the demands of industry. According to Dulles:

> At the century's end, New York reported half as many Italians as Naples, as many Germans as Hamburg, as many Jews as Warsaw, and twice as many Irish as Dublin. The foreign-born in Chicago exceeded its total population of a decade earlier. Its busy streets were crowded with Germans, Swedes, Norwegians, Italians, Poles, Lithuanians, Hungarians, and Slovenes. And, in varying degrees, much the same could be said of other urban centers from Boston to St. Louis.[8]

Whole families were crowded into dark, damp, poorly ventilated rooms—often with no outside windows—which opened only onto sunless shafts. Plumbing facilities were antiquated or nonexistent and, of necessity, shared by many. Poorly constructed, overcrowded tenements, difficult to reach, made the danger of devastating fires imminent, and the ominous clanging firetruck was a frequent visitor. The sanitary and health conditions were intolerable. Tuberculosis, diphtheria, and venereal diseases were just a few of the many com-municable diseases which were rampant. Poverty, overcrowding, and lack of recreational facilities furnished an environment in which crime and delinquency flourished. Public health measures were emi-nently inadequate to cope with such overwhelming problems. A growing concern about the environment in which people were living and the responsibility of the community for the protection of the individual was beginning to be apparent everywhere. Numerous books and articles graphically describing the intolerable living and working conditions of the people in the slums made their appear-ance. Publishing houses multiplied. The ranks of those concerned increased, fed by a growing middle class and a better educated and informed public. Reform groups organized and flourished. Many of these directed their energies toward the social and health fields.

Equally as bad as the slum environment were the working condi-tions. Men, women, and children, separately and as family units, labored in dark, crowded, poorly ventilated shops and factories 10 to

[8] Dulles, *op. cit.*, p. 90.

12 hours a day, for 6 days a week—all for less than a living wage. It is difficult for us to understand why the situation was tolerated as long as it was. It was probably due to the fact that America was thought to be a land of promise and opportunity. A feeling of optimism prevailed. Anything was within the realm of possibility, if not for the parents, perhaps for the children. The very struggle for life itself was worth the rewards which might be ahead. Many immigrants were able to save money, buy small businesses, and improve their living and working conditions. The desire of these individuals to retain their freedom, to grasp any opportunity which might present itself, may account for the fact that sporadic attempts toward organization of workers into labor unions failed, for the most part, during this period.

The population expanded by leaps and bounds, doubled between 1870 and 1890, and by 1900 was 76,303,387.[9] By this time immigration had contributed 20 million newcomers.[10] In spite of the problems of the poor, America was predominantly a middle-class society, and this was expanding. Class structure was not rigid, and aspirations for upward mobility were high and often realized. The standard of living was improving, and families with higher incomes and better transportation were beginning to move out of the crowded cities and settle in the suburbs. In sharp contrast to the grinding poverty of some was the tremendous wealth of a small but increasing segment of the population. Men such as Andrew Carnegie, who exemplified the rags-to-riches heroes, felt they owed something to America for their good fortunes. They gave huge sums to charity based on the philosophy of helping those who wished to help themselves. Thus, public philanthropy was begun by those men who had been able to make a great deal of money by utilizing the fruits of society and who wished to give back to society a portion of their money and opportunity.

Education

The concept of the value of education for all in a free society had been built into the very fabric of American life and was taking hold. Education gave hope and possibility for individ-

---

[9]Bureau of the Census, *op. cit.*, p. 55.
[10]Hacker, L. M., and Kendrick, B. B. *The United States Since 1865*. New York, F. S. Crofts and Company, 1935, p. 139.

ual advancement, for solutions of society's complex problems, and for acquisition of new knowledge applicable to business and industry. The task of providing education for such a polyglot people seemed almost insurmountable. Most of the wealthy were educated privately, many of the poor, not at all. Middle-class children attended good and bad, large and small, public and private schools. Agitation for free public education persisted and grew. The federal government was supportive but left to the states the job of overseeing and regulating this heterogeneous system of education. By 1900 the average American had 1046 days of school, or more than twelve times as much as his great-grandfather.[11] Between 1870 and 1900 the number of high schools rose from 500 to 6,000.[12] However, less than 10 percent of the population reached high school, and less than 1 percent went to college.[13]

Reform was not limited to grammar and secondary school education. Well-established men's private colleges in the East were trying to create some sort of order out of the new conditions. They were tackling the problem of shaping an educational plan that would be as meaningful for their students as classical education had been for earlier students. They began to study and to revise their curricula, to de-emphasize preparation for the clergy, and to expand offerings in the humanities and in the sciences. State universities appeared in the West and made higher education available for both men and women. The western tradition of educating boys and girls together in grammar and high school carried over to university education.

There was a great difference of opinion, and controversy, over higher education for women. Some critics believed that sustained brain activity would drain away strength from child-bearing ability; college women desiring children would be incapable of safe and sound motherhood; and college education would ruin a girl's body instincts and unsex her. The severest critics, nevertheless, agreed that they would rather have educated than uneducated women teach their children. In spite of controversy educational opportunities for women increased. Nothing could really have stopped it. The time was ripe and there were always people ready and eager to take up the challenge. Private women's colleges developed in the East where there was the tradition of private men's colleges. By June, 1899,

[11]Ross, E. A. *Changing America.* New York, The Century Company, 1919, p. 6.
[12]Dulles, *op. cit.,* p. 104.
[13]Hill, H. W., *The New Public Health.* New York, The Macmillan Company, 1916, p. 30.

14,824 women had earned a bachelor's degree. This was the largest number of educated women in any country in the world. [14]

In 1876 the first graduate school was established at Johns Hopkins University. By 1900 graduate education was becoming increasingly important, and was established, for the most part, within the graduate schools of the larger universities. Graduate professional education in law, medicine, theology, dentistry, and veterinary medicine increased. The percentage of women admitted to these schools showed a greater increase than that of men.

Many factors contributed to the development of higher education for both men and women. Not the least of these were the philosophy of individualism and the noninterfering role of the government. Men who had become wealthy as a result of the industrial revolution found a fruitful and satisfying outlet for their philanthropy in colleges and universities. By contributing to higher education they were also influencing the improvement of educational opportunities for their sons. The resources of a growing body of alumni also added to educational and financial support. High value was placed on scientific knowledge and its importance to technology, without which industrialization could not have occurred.

Women

Perhaps one of the greatest changes occurred during this period in the status and role of women. The results of the industrial revolution, such as the development of the typewriter and need for clerical help, opened up new possibilities for women to work outside the home and to secure some measure of economic independence. The unquenchable thirst of the people for more goods created a constant need for workers to produce them, and many women wishing to supplement their family's income (inadequate because of low wages) moved into these jobs. By and large these women worked long hours and had little time or energy left over to become involved in the general ferment over women's rights.

As a result of technical advances and an abundant supply of domestic help, a growing number of women in the upper and middle income levels were relieved of much of their household drudgery. Because of their social position work outside the home was frowned

[14]Butler, N. M., ed. *Education in the United States*, Vols. I and II. Albany, N. Y., J. B. Lyon Company, 1900, p. 352.

upon, even though they were living in the midst of a bustling society in which work was considered a virtue. Some of these women exemplified the genteel, frail woman whose main mission in life was to amuse her husband. These were usually the ones who became the leaders and participants in the gay society of the times. Others were not satisfied with this role and became involved in a variety of educational, health, social, and political reforms.

As the number of women with higher education grew, their influence was felt in many areas. Improved education for teachers was raising the level of instruction in public schools. Women authors were becoming abundant. Women participated in public debates and gave lectures on a variety of subjects. Womens' organizations sprang up, and in 1889 the Federation of Women's Clubs was established. As the level of education improved and as the members became more aware of the society in which they lived, the programs of these organizations expanded and many became powerful forces in social and political reform.

The mobility of the population brought about a marked change in family life. Relatives who had previously lived in proximity to one another found themselves separated and living in unfamiliar surroundings. The authoritarian position of the husband and father was weakened as the wife assumed more responsibility for the caring and rearing of children, as well as for the economic support of the family. The birth rate was decreasing and divorce was on the rise.

The growing militancy of women for their right to vote gained momentous proportions. By 1900 women were voting in many local elections, and four western states had given equal suffrage to women.[15]

The increasing independence and growing participation of women in all facets of society were frowned upon by the majority of men and a large number of women. Many of the ills of society, such as the breakup of families, illegitimacy, the juvenile crime rate, and the increase in venereal disease were blamed on the fact that women were not at home where they belonged.

Nursing

Some of the women who had been involved in the Civil War had become friends with Florence Nightingale and had gone to England to observe the developments in the training school for

[15] Dulles, *op. cit.*, p. 187.

nurses which she had established. Others began corresponding with her and were learning more about her philosophy of nursing. Her book, *Notes on Nursing*, had become more readily available to readers in the United States with the improved transportation, and many were using some of her methods in nursing their own family members. Some of the Ladies Aid Societies that were established during the War had continued as organized groups and were involved in various philanthropic and charitable works. One of these, the State Charities Aid Association of New York, sponsored a study in 1872 of the care of patients at Bellevue Hospital. The deplorable state of the patients and the poor care they were receiving appalled and shocked the members. The Association was instrumental in bringing these intolerable conditions to the attention of the public. At the same time some of the technologic advances, such as the development of the sphygmomanometer and the hypodermic, were changing medical and nursing practices. The introduction of asepsis, new surgical techniques, and improved preoperative and postoperative care were demanding better prepared personnel and a new relationship between doctors and nurses. Physicians were becoming more and more concerned about the care their patients were receiving, and some gave individual and group instruction to the women who were nursing them. Women physicians were increasing in number and, because of the opposition against them, were particularly anxious to prove their worth. Some were personally involved in improving nursing care for their patients. In 1867 Dr. Marie Zakrzewska, who was professor of obstetrics at the New England Female Medical College in Boston, initiated a nursing program at the New England Hospital for Women and Children. This program later developed under the direction of Dr. Susan Dimock. Linda Richards successfully completed the program and received a diploma in 1872. She is often referred to as the first trained nurse in the United States.

A year later the first three modern training schools for nurses were established—one at Bellevue Hospital, one at New Haven Hospital, and the other at the Massachusetts General Hospital. Each of these schools, using the model developed by Florence Nightingale, was established by lay groups who were financially independent of the hospital. However, due to lack of funds and strong opposition from the medical profession, they succumbed early to financial control by the hospital. Thus, the pattern of hospital control of nursing was established, and from then on training schools emerged at the whim of the individual hospitals.

There was considerable opposition from many sources to the new system of training schools for nurses, and fear was expressed that the nurses would be taught too much and think they knew more than the physicians. There was also apprehension that better-educated women would not enter the nursing schools and, if they did, would become disillusioned and leave nursing after they had been trained. However, it soon became evident that patients received better care when pupil nurses were available, that the death rate of patients in hospitals where there were pupils decreased, and that pupils were a cheap source of labor. As a result new hospitals developed, and the number of training schools for nurses increased by leaps and bounds.

The early schools of nursing grew up in a haphazard individualistic way with each hospital a law unto itself. There were no uniform admission standards, and pupils with eighth-grade education were taught together with college graduates. The length of the courses varied from 1 to 2 years. Pupils worked from 10 to 12 or more hours each day. There was no standard curriculum pattern, and classes were held irregularly in addition to the long work day. Militarylike discipline prevailed with absolute obedience to the physician. Pupils lived in nurses' homes set up by the hospital and were socially isolated from the outside world. The overwhelming majority of the graduates went into private nursing, usually on a 24-hour-a-day basis. The hospitals were staffed entirely by pupil nurses, and the employment of staff nurses in the hospital was not even considered. The schools were organized to carry on the work of the hospitals and not to educate nurses.

In spite of these conditions women from the middle and upper income groups enrolled in the nursing schools, and there was no problem of recruitment. Apparently, the opportunity to care for the sick provided these women with a satisfying outlet for the idealism and humanitarianism so characteristic of nursing and the times. Nursing also opened up a whole new occupation for women whose opportunities had previously been limited primarily to teaching.

At the same time that nursing was getting deeper and deeper into the apprenticeship type of education, medical education was going in the opposite direction and beginning to give up the apprenticeship system. There was a movement toward medical schools becoming fully independent of the hospitals in which their students had experience, and setting up university hospitals under their own control.

By 1893 there were 225 schools of nursing,[16] and the number was growing. This rapid proliferation made it imperative that some common education standards be developed if nursing were to become a profession. Nursing, too, had women of imagination and vision who were ready and willing to take up the challenge. One of the outstanding ones was Isabel Hampton (Robb). She exemplified the eminent women who were the leaders in many of the contemporary social, educational, health, and political endeavors. She had a background of private school education, had received an upbringing characteristic of middle- and upper-class society, and had taught school before entering nursing. It was largely through her leadership that in 1893 the Society of Superintendents of Training Schools of Nurses of the United States and Canada was organized. According to Roberts:

> The primary purposes of the new society were to advance the best interest of the nursing profession by establishing and maintaining a universal standard of training, and by promoting fellowship among its members by meetings, papers, and discussions on nursing subjects and by interchange of opinions.[17]

This organization was later to become the National League for Nursing Education. The membership consisted primarily of administrators and directors of schools of nursing.

Two years later the Nurses' Associated Alumnae Association of the United States and Canada, which later became the American Nurses' Association, was organized. It opened its membership to all alumnae of training schools for nurses. It stated that:

> The objects of this Association shall be to strengthen the union of nursing organizations; to elevate nursing education; to promote ethical standards in all the relations of the nursing profession.[18]

With the establishment of these two organizations, nursing had taken a giant step toward becoming a profession. There was now a medium by which nurses could develop criteria and standards for nursing practice and nursing education, could develop a code of ethics, and could meet together to discuss common problems and share new techniques and developments.

[16]Shyrock, H. *The History of Nursing.* Philadelphia, W. B. Saunders Company, 1959, p. 300.
[17]Roberts, M. M. *American Nursing.* New York, The Macmillan Company, 1954, p. 25.
[18]Nurses' Associated Alumnae of the United States. Minutes of Proceedings Fifth Annual Convention, Chicago, May 1, 2, and 3, 1902. *Amer. J. Nurs.*, 2:766, July 1902.

Public Health Nursing   It was not until 1886, after
the value of organized nursing
care in the hospitals and the
benefit of private nursing to
patients in their own homes had been demonstrated, that organized
district nursing developed. It was because of the success of private
nursing to patients in the upper and middle income levels that
questions were raised about how to bring a similar type of service to
the poor. At the same time application of the germ theory was laying
the groundwork for control of communicable disease. Poverty was
beginning to be considered a result of social maladjustment; and
there was a belief that the benefits of medicine and nursing should be
available equally to the poor and the rich.

There had been sporadic attempts for many years to provide some
nursing care to the sick poor in their homes. In many instances
women had been employed by churches, guilds, settlement houses,
dispensaries, and other charitable organizations to go into the home
of the sick persons who were connected with the particular organization. However, these attempts, though laudable in their purposes,
were not too successful. The women who were employed were not
necessarily trained and did not always know how to give nursing care
in the home, particularly when they were confronted with the many
other problems of the people who lived in the slums. Nursing was
often secondary to other purposes for visiting, and it was not clear
what nursing care in the homes really included. Also, this early
nursing service was mixed with charity and almsgiving, with bringing
a religious message to the family, with being only a follow-up of the
doctor's orders to the patient, and with being associated with a free
dispensary. Nursing was not a primary focus for visiting, and the
availability of nursing services to all the people in the community
was not a part of these early attempts.

The first organized district nursing began in 1886, and at first,
according to Jacques,[19] the nurses merely followed the physicians'
orders, gave some treatments, and recorded the temperature and
pulse. However, this was much more than the patient had previously
received, and the physician, patient, and family all looked upon this
amount of professional care as a great advancement. The nurses very
soon realized that because they were in the home for only a short

[19]Jacques, M. *District Nursing*. New York, The Macmillan Company, 1911, pp. 6-12.

time, in contrast to the private duty nurse, someone had to be taught to take care of the patient between the nurses' visits. Instruction to families about how to care for the patient naturally included personal hygiene, sanitary measures of the sick room, and aspects of healthful living for the entire family. Thus, almost from the very beginning, teaching and prevention became important functions of the district nurse.

The first district nursing associations, one in Boston and one in Philadelphia, were formed in the same year. Each developed in a different way and without any relationship to the other. However, both were organized by women who were inspired by the work of William Rathbone in England and who had investigated the organization of district nursing in Liverpool. In Boston two socially conscious women approached the Women's Education Association to support the work of a district nurse. They had to convince the Association that district nursing related mainly to education, in order for its sponsorship to be consistent with the other educational efforts of the Association. Thus, the title Instructive District Nursing was coined. The group then met with persons in the Boston Dispensary, which was providing free medical care to the sick poor and had divided the city into dispensary districts, to discuss how the two groups could work together. As a result, in February of 1886, one nurse was employed to work in one dispensary district. It was not long before other nurses were employed for the other districts. The nurse in each district was assigned to a physician and was responsible for carrying out medical orders. Sometimes the doctor and nurse would visit a patient together. The patients were not charged any fee for the service. Supervision was given by two lay managers of the association who were assigned to each district. It was not until 1900 that a nurse was employed to oversee the work and to supervise the nurses.

It was not long before the value of the work was well recognized, and in 1888 the Instructive District Nursing Association was incorporated and became an independent voluntary agency. The objects were:

1. To provide and support thoroughly trained nurses, who, acting under the immediate direction of the out-patient physician of the Boston Dispensary, shall care for the sick poor in their own homes instead of in hospitals.

2. By precept and example to give such instruction to the families which they are called upon to visit as shall enable them henceforth to

take better care of themselves and their neighbors by observing the rules of wholesome living and by practicing the simple arts of domestic nursing.[20]

Probably the emphasis on teaching of the Boston organization was due in part to its early sponsorship by the Women's Education Association. However, the teaching function of the nurse had been stressed by Florence Nightingale and was one of the strengths of the early organizations.

At the same time that the work was being developed in Boston, a group of prominent women in Philadelphia, who had also been inspired by William Rathbone's work, organized and employed a nurse to give nursing to the sick at home. They were not sponsored or affiliated with any other group and at first had trouble finding patients. They only had $100.00 with which to start their venture and decided very early to charge the patients for the cost of the carfare of the nurse. It soon became evident, as the service became better known, that patients other than just the sick poor needed and wanted nursing service from the district nurse. As a result, they decided to charge the patient for the cost of the nursing visit. The Visiting Nurse Society of Philadelphia was incorporated in 1887. The purpose was "to furnish visiting nurses to those otherwise unable to secure skilled attendance in time of sickness, to teach cleanliness and proper care of the sick."[21] At the end of the first year a nurse was employed to direct the service and to supervise the nurses.

In this period it was becoming increasingly popular for persons interested in charitable and philanthropic work to band together and form settlements or settlement houses in the slums of the larger cities. Some of the groups were sponsored by universities, and graduate students and their wives lived in the settlement houses which became the base of their operations. Others were composed of groups of men and women who were concerned about the plight of the poor and felt they could contribute most to understanding and alleviating some of their miseries by living among the people and becoming intimately involved in their everyday problems. Activities and programs of all kinds were developed in the settlement houses to meet the needs of the people in the neighborhoods in which the

[20]Brainard, A. M. *Evolution of Public Health Nursing.* Philadelphia, W. B. Saunders Company, 1922, p. 207.
[21]*Ibid.*, p. 219.

houses were established. Many of the leaders in the settlement house movement became very active in bringing to the attention of the public the miserable conditions of the lives of the poor, and took leadership in agitating for social legislation to change conditions.

In 1893 Lillian Wald and her friend Mary Brewster, both trained nurses and wealthy in their own right, launched the district nursing service for the sick poor in New York. They moved into the neighborhood because they felt they would be more readily available to the people and would be looked upon as friends and neighbors. They became interested in all aspects of the community and were instrumental in establishing the Henry Street Settlement House. Its program included many activities for the people in the community; however, nursing always remained one of the major activities. From the inception of the nursing program the nurses were not identified with any one physician, with a free dispensary, or with a religious group. The patients were always charged fees according to their ability to pay. Calls were received from all physicians as well as from the people themselves, and the nurses maintained strict professional relationships with the physicians and the patients. Many of these ideas were revolutionary and laid the basis for a whole new relationship between the patient and the nurse. From the beginning nursing was under the supervision of nurses. Lillian Wald also believed that nursing should be aligned with the official health agency, and made arrangements with the health department for the nurses to wear an insignia which signified they were under the auspices of the board of health.

It was Lillian Wald who first used the term *public health nurse* and she describes her reason as follows:

> We called our enterprise "public health nursing." Our basic idea was that the nurse's peculiar introduction to the patient and her organic relationship with the neighborhood should constitute the starting point for a universal service to the region. Our purpose was in no sense to establish an isolated undertaking. We planned to utilize, as well as to be implemented by, all agencies and groups of whatever creed which were working for social betterment, private as well as municipal. Our scheme was to be motivated by a vital sense of the interrelation of all these forces. For this reason we considered ourselves best described by the term "public health nurses."[22]

[22]Wales, M. *The Public Health Nurse in Action.* New York, The Macmillan Company, 1941, Forward, p. xi.

At about the same time in Los Angeles a group of women in another settlement, called the College Settlement, appealed to the City Council for a monthly allowance for the salary of a district nurse who would give nursing care to the sick poor in their homes. The City Council agreed, and in 1898 the first nurse paid for by public funds started work under the direction of the Committee of Women in the College Settlement.

By 1900, there were twenty district nursing organizations employing 200 nurses.[23] Most were in the large cities, but some were also in the smaller communities. Each developed in its own way with no uniformity in organizational structure, sponsor, methods, records, hours of work, policies, finances, or services. This approach, similar to that of other endeavors in the United States, was consistent with the philosophy of individualism that was prevalent at that time. The federal government still maintained its laissez faire attitude and had not as yet assumed any responsibility for the overall health of the people. In contrast, in England where district nursing was also a voluntary movement, a centralized, voluntary, uniform system of organization was being developed.

In spite of the diversity of district nursing organizations in the United States, the groundwork was being laid for their further expansion and development. Some of the basic principles of public health nursing were becoming apparent. It was increasingly evident that nursing should be available to all who were sick, regardless of ability to pay or religious affiliation; a definite distinction was being made between nursing and almsgiving; nurses were beginning to recognize the importance of keeping records; professional relationships between the doctor and nurse were carefully guarded and maintained; and the importance of cooperation with other groups in the community was being stressed in order to provide the best care to the patient. It was recognized that district nurses needed more preparation than they received in hospital programs.

Summary

In any society, at any point in time, there are certain pervasive ideas and beliefs which people hold as values and which strongly influence decisions which they will make about those

[23]Shyrock, *op. cit.*, p. 298.

things which affect their very way of life. Some of the overriding ideas in the post-Civil War period were:

> America was a land of opportunity, and anything was possible.
>
> Hard work was worth the effort and would pay off—if not in the present, then certainly in the future.
>
> This was a free country, a haven for everyone, and the doors would be open for those who wished to enter.
>
> Those whom the country had favored with good fortune should show their gratitude by helping those who were less fortunate.
>
> Public education was important if a free society was to grow and prosper.
>
> Higher education was important for men.
>
> Women's place was in the home for the bearing and rearing of children.
>
> Individualism was paramount, and the role of the government was to make individualism possible.
>
> The community was not responsible for the welfare of its people.

This was a period of rapid growth and progress, and there were many people who had different dreams and ideas for this young country. Many felt that:

> Women should have more independence and freedom, a greater voice in decision making, and equal opportunity for higher education.
>
> Those concerned about problems of real social import, such as unhealthy slum conditions, poor environment, and deplorable care in hospitals, should organize and do something to change the situation.

Expansion of the railroads, industrialization, developments in science and technology, improved communication, progress in education, and changes in the role of women challenged many of the generally accepted beliefs of the times and influenced the ideas of many about the directions of America for the future. By the end of the period, there was:

> More acceptance of the value of higher education for women, with increasing numbers of women enrolled in colleges and universities.
>
> More recognition of the rights of women and their potential contribution to society. Women were demonstrating leadership and organizational ability and were seeking opportunities outside of the home.
>
> A growing dream that the fruits of knowledge, industrialization, science, and technology should be available to everyone. This was beginning to happen.

Realization that the community could do something about its problems. A reform movement which was to later grow and flourish had already begun.

The development of nursing and district nursing in this period was an inevitable outgrowth of the times and all the forces that were being generated in society. It is impossible to separate out any one of the developments as generating the most important forces as it was a combination of the total. Perhaps nursing was an idea whose time had come. The industrial revolution, which was improving the quality of life for many, was also helping to pinpoint the discrepancies between the "haves" and the "have-nots." At the same time people were learning more about the increasing plight of the poor as wave after wave of immigrants settled in the slums of cities. A social consciousness which was characterized by idealism and humanitarianism was gaining momentum among various groups of people, particularly the better-educated women. This idealism and humanitarianism was the overriding impetus contributing to the development of nursing. Nursing also had great appeal to women who were rebelling against a restrictive society which said women's place was in the home. A whole new era for women was developing, and nursing speeded this development by providing a new occupation in which women from all segments of society could participate. Caring for the sick was a tangible expression of one's humanitarianism and tended to give one a sense of satisfaction or fulfillment. The harder one worked, the more she could contribute to the easing of suffering of others. Thus, the stage was set for all kinds of exploitation of nurses. Hard work, militarylike discipline, social isolation, and little or no education other than what was learned on the job were accepted without question. The overriding mission was service to the sick, and the other factors were only tangential to that mission. Protection of the woman by the man was a pervasive theme of the times, so the domination of nursing by medicine was a natural outgrowth.

Interested citizen groups spearheaded the development of both hospital nursing and district nursing. However, as hospital nursing became more and more dominated by physicians, the role of the citizen diminished. On the other hand, the development of district nursing was contingent from the beginning on citizen participation. Citizen groups were responsible for organizing the service, for policies governing the organization, for interpreting to the community what the nurses could do—in other words, doing everything they could to make it possible for the nurse to use her knowledge and skill in taking care of the sick poor in their own homes. In many instances the citizen groups consisted of wealthy women who were seeking a way to do good, and district nursing provided this outlet. Unfortunately, this lady-bountiful attitude also carried over in their relationships with the nurses whom they employed, and this often hampered the development of a viable partnership between the nurses and the lay groups. However, the seeds were being sown, and a model of lay and professional collaboration was evolving. District nursing was also moving in different directions from hospital nursing in other areas. Because district nurses were less isolated from the people and their day-by-day problems, they soon recognized that nurses needed more education to understand these problems and how to help the people cope with them. The sick poor who lived in the slums of the larger cities were their main focus, but by the end of the period this emphasis was beginning to shift. There was some thinking that district nursing should be available to everyone. Those who could pay for the service should do so, but no one should be refused service because of inability to pay.

As was mentioned earlier, the development of nursing and district nursing during this period was inevitable. The impact of this development had far-reaching effects. Probably the most important was on the role of women and their place in society. Nursing was not only a whole new occupation for women, but it generated the development of other occupations in which women could participate.

On the other hand, the germination of nursing in the hospital with the long hours and heavy emphasis on service sapped the energy of the nurses and left them little time to think about the direction nursing should take. Thus, the apprenticeship system of education for nursing became entrenched, and the nurse as the handmaiden of the physician was generally accepted. By the end of the period, however, some nurses were challenging these assumptions, and agitation was beginning for better education and for some control of the quality of nursing practice.

REFERENCES

Allen, F. L. The Big Change. New York, Harper and Brothers, 1952.
American Public Health Association. A Half Century of Public Health — Jubilee

Historical Volume of the American Public Health Association. Lynn, Mass., The Nichols Press, 1921.

Babbidge, H. D., and Rosenzweig, R. M. The Federal Interest in Higher Education. New York, McGraw-Hill Company, Inc., 1962.

Blum, J. M. The Promise of America. Cambridge, Mass., Houghton Mifflin Company, 1966.

Brainard, A. M. Evolution of Public Health Nursing. Philadelphia, W. B. Saunders Company, 1922.

———— Organization of Public Health Nursing. New York, The Macmillan Company, 1919.

Brockett, L. P. Woman: Her Rights, Wrongs, Privileges, and Responsibilities. Hartford, L. Stebbins, 1869.

———— and Vaughan, M. C. Woman's Work in the Civil War: A Record of Heroism, Patriotism, and Patience. Rochester, N. Y., Curran, 1867.

Brooks, V. W. Three Essays on America. New York, E. P. Dutton and Company, 1934.

Bryson, L. Facing the Future's Risks. New York, Harper and Brothers, 1953.

Bureau of the Census. A Century of Population Growth: 1790-1900. Washington, D.C., Government Printing Office, 1909.

Butler, N. M., ed. Education in the United States, Vols. I and II. Albany, N. Y., J. B. Lyon Company, 1900.

Calhoun, A. W. A Social History of the American Family, Vol. III. Cleveland, The Arthur E. Clark Company, 1919.

Dawson, C. The Crisis of Western Education. New York, Sheed and Ward, 1961.

DeVane, W. C. Higher Education in Twentieth Century America. Cambridge, Mass., Harvard University Press, 1965.

Dock, L. A Short History of Nursing, 2nd ed. New York, G. P. Putnam's Sons, 1925.

Dolan, J. Goodnow's History of Nursing, 11th ed. Philadelphia, W. B. Saunders Company, 1963.

Dowd, D. F. Modern Economic Problems in Historical Perspective. Boston, D. C. Heath and Company, 1962.

Dulles, F. R. The United States Since 1865. Ann Arbor, The University of Michigan Press, 1959.

Fraser, G. W. An Introduction to the Study of Education. New York, Harper and Brothers, 1951.

Gardner, M. S. Public Health Nursing. New York, The Macmillan Company, 1916.

Garrison, F. H. History of Medicine. Philadelphia, W. B. Saunders Company, 1929.

Greenbie, M. B. Lincoln's Daughters of Mercy. New York, G. P. Putnam's Sons, 1944.

Hacker, L. M. The Triumph of American Capitalism. New York, Simon and Schuster, 1940.

———— and Kendrick, B. B. The United States Since 1865. New York, F. S. Crofts and Company, 1935.

Hamburg, D. Principles of a Growing Economy. New York, W. W. Norton and Company, 1961.

Handlin, O. The Americans. Boston, Little, Brown and Company, 1963.

———— Chance or Destiny. Boston, Little, Brown and Company, 1955.

———— This Was America. London, Oxford University Press, 1949.

Hill, H. W. The New Public Health. New York, The Macmillan Company, 1916.

Jacques, M. District Nursing. New York, The Macmillan Company, 1911.

Jamieson, E. M. Trends in Nursing History. Philadelphia, W. B. Saunders Company, 1960.

Kaul. A. N. The American Vision. New Haven, Yale University Press, 1963.

Kraus, M. The United States to 1965. Ann Arbor, The University of Michigan Press, 1959.

Miyakawa, T. S. Protestants and Pioneers. Chicago, University of Chicago Press, 1964.

Merry, E. J., and Iris, D. I. District Nursing, 2nd ed. London, Bailliere Tindall and Cox, 1955.

Morgan, H. W., ed. The Gilded Age. Syracuse, Syracuse University Press, 1963.

Nurses' Associated Alumnae of the United States. Minutes of Proceedings Fifth Annual Convention, Chicago, May 1, 2, and 3, 1902. Amer. J. Nurs., 2:745-898, July 1902.

Nutting, M. A. A Sound Educational Economic Basis for Schools of Nursing and Other Addresses. New York, G. P. Putnam's Sons, 1926.

———— Education Status of Nursing. U. S. Bureau of Education Bulletin, No. 7. Washington, D. C., Government Printing Office, 1912.

Richards, L. Reminiscences of Linda Richards, America's First Trained Nurse. Boston, Whitcomb and Barrows, 1911.

Riis, J. The Battle With the Slums. New York, The Macmillan Company, 1902.

Robb, I. H. Educational Standards for Nurses. 1907.

Roberts, M. M. American Nursing. New York, The Macmillan Company, 1954.

Ross, E. A. Changing America. New York, The Century Company, 1919.

Shyrock, R. H. The History of Nursing. Philadelphia, W. B. Saunders Company, 1959.

Smillie, W. G. Public Health—Its Promise for the Future. New York, The Macmillan Company, 1955.

———— and Kilbourne, E. D. Preventive Medicine and Public Health. New York, The Macmillan Company, 1963.

Thomson, W. G. Training Schools for Nurses. New York, G. P. Putnam's Sons, 1883.

Wald, L. D. Windows on Henry Street. Boston, Little, Brown and Company, 1954.

———— The House on Henry Street. New York, Henry Holt and Company, 1938.

Wales, M. The Public Health Nurse in Action. New York, The Macmillan Company, 1941.

Weeks-Shaw, C. A. Text Book of Nursing. New York, D. Appleton and Company, 1902.

Winslow, C.-E. A., Smillie, W. G., Doull, J. A., and Gordon, J. E. In F. H. Top, ed. The History of American Epidemiology. St. Louis, The C. V. Mosby Company, 1952.

Woods, R. A. The Poor in Great Cities—Their Problems and What Is Doing to Solve Them. New York, Charles Scribner's Sons, 1895.

Worcester, A. Nurses For Our Neighbors. Boston, Houghton Mifflin Company, 1914.

CHAPTER 2

The Period From 1900 to the New Deal

Overview

By the turn of the century America was a young united nation endowed with the necessary ingredients for rapid growth and development. During the next 35 years there was phenomenal expansion in transportation, industrialization, and public education. It was a period in which nursing grew in stature, became a respected occupation for women, and demonstrated its real potential for professionalism. It was a time of study, experimentation, and evaluation, and of concern for quality of both nursing practice and education. Preparation of some nurses within institutions of higher education became a reality, made possible by the quality of leadership in nursing and the interest and support of foundations and philanthropists. The concept of the responsibility of the community for the health of its citizens became an accepted part of public health. The time was right for the phenomenal growth of public health nursing.

Social consciousness invaded every aspect of life. Voluntary agencies proliferated. The first part of the century was marked by feverish activity for social and legislative reform that would benefit all the people, instead of just a privileged few. This activity came to a halt at the time of the First World War. During the twenties people became preoccupied with enjoying the good things of life, and the prewar reform spirit was not revitalized. The end of the period was marked by a great depression which had immeasurable influence on all Americans and their way of life. It sounded the death knell to rugged individualism, proved that voluntary organizations were no longer able to meet the overwhelming social and health needs of the people, and made it imperative that the government assume its constitutional responsibility for the general welfare.

Transportation

The automobile was to this period what the railroad had been to the preceding one. In 1900 there were only 13,824 cars in the United States.[1] They were considered status symbols which only the wealthy could afford. This was true, at least until 1908 when Henry Ford developed the Model-T and brought automobile ownership within the reach of everyone. In 1914 he introduced the assembly line in the production of his car. This method of mass production was destined to revolutionize transportation and the entire character of American society. The basis of the assembly line was that mass production of cars would lower the cost of each one and reduce the price to the buyer. The profit on an individual car would be small, but because of the larger number sold, the total profit would be large. In order for the assembly line to function successfully, each worker had to become competent in only one small phase of the total production process. By 1915 there were more than 2,225,000 registered automobiles,[2] and they were well on the way to becoming a necessity for the modern way of life.

After the war the automobile was no longer considered a luxury but an indispensable part of life. The Model-T became a symbol of

[1] Allen, F. L. *The Big Change.* New York, Harper and Brothers, 1952, p. 124.
[2] Morris, L. D. *Not So Long Ago.* New York, Random House, 1949, p. 324.

democracy in which everyone could afford to own a car, thus reducing the social distance between the upper and lower income groups. Paved roads and highways increased and were spurred by the Federal Highways Act of 1921 which gave money to the states on a matching basis for the construction of certain highways. Filling stations and garages became commonplace. The isolation of the farmer ended, and dependence on the railroads lessened. Provincialism decreased as people traveled from one section of the country to another. Tourist homes, camp grounds, and hot dog stands mushroomed along well-traveled highways. Many people moved to the suburbs and commuted to work. Traffic congestion and parking problems grew. Automobile accidents increased in proportion to car ownership. In contrast to the pessimistic reaction to the appearance of the automobile, President Hoover's Committee on Social Trends reported "that no invention of such far-reaching importance was ever diffused with such rapidity, or so quickly exerted influence that ramified through the normal culture, transforming even habits of thought and language."[3]

By 1935, the number had risen to 3,273,874 passenger cars, and 697,367 trucks and buses for a total of 3,971,241.[4] The railroads were beginning to feel the bite of competition.

Air travel developed slowly and did not reach maturity until after 1935. The Wright brothers, in 1903, had carried out the first successful experiment with the airplane, but this event went almost unnoticed. It was not until after World War I that aviation became a commercial venture and was subsidized by the government for mail service. Delivery of mail by air was as important to this period as it was by continental railroad in 1869. By 1934 aviation had expanded with 24 American airlines carrying one-half million passengers over 51,000 miles of established air routes.[5]

Industrialization and Technology

At the beginning of the century industry had become big business, and giant corporations, monopolies, and trusts were dominating the economy. The laissez faire attitude of the

[3] *Ibid.*, p. 284.
[4] Rae, J. B. *The American Automobile.* Chicago, University of Chicago Press, 1965, p. 238.
[5] Dulles, F. *The United States Since 1865.* Ann Arbor, The University of Michigan Press, 1959, p. 311.

government as well as some of the decisions of the Supreme Court favored the practices of the industrial giants. Several states had passed legislation in an attempt to exert some control but, as had happened similarly in the earlier period with the development of railroad companies, the state laws were geared to the interests of the individual states and often were unrelated to the overall needs of the country. However, the general public was becoming more aware of the effect of the practices of big business on the country as a whole and was beginning to rebel and to agitate for stronger government control in the interest of the general welfare. The government was forced to come to grips with some of the hard-core problems of industrialization and in 1914 passed the Clayton Act which attempted to regulate monopolistic practices and to protect the individual consumer.

Unionization of labor was gaining momentum, but there was no unified movement and only token support by the government. Some gains were being made in specialized areas, but for the most part poor working conditions, low pay, long hours of work, and the employment of women and children prevailed. The reform spirit, so prevalent in the first part of the century, had embraced the plight of workers and had been instrumental in the passage of some state legislation which favored them. However, some of these laws were declared unconstitutional by the Supreme Court. The most revolutionary change in favor of the workers was made by Henry Ford when in 1914 he shocked the world by raising the wages from $2.50 for a 9-hour day to $5.00 for an 8-hour day. At the same time the price of his car went down from $950.00 in 1909 to $290.00 in 1924.[6]

After the war the technical know-how and the ingenuity of the American people, plus the assembly-line principle of mass production, fed the healthy and growing industrial system, and the economy flourished. All sorts of consumer goods, appliances, and gadgets appeared on the market and were available to everyone in all walks of life. The acquisition of the same products by people of different socioeconomic levels tended to blur the sharp lines of distinction between the rich and the poor and to stabilize and to universalize the culture.

The expansion of the movies and the radio also contributed to a

[6]Mowry, F. *The Urban Nation 1920-1960.* New York, Hill and Wang, 1965, p. 13.

more common culture. Moving pictures, which had been developed prior to the war, became a major industry in the twenties and a power for influencing public opinion. The impact of the movies was incalculable—they were the major source of entertainment and of ideas about life in general. Movie stars became the leaders, opinion makers, and pacesetters in society. The fashions, manners, morals, and ways of living depicted in the movies exerted their influence in every walk of life.

Population and Immigration

The population in 1900 was 75.9 million and the life expectancy at birth about 50 years. Within the next 25 years the population had increased to approximately 114 million, and life expectancy at birth had risen to 60 years for women and about 58 for men.[7]

Immigrants continued to pour into the country with approximately one million admitted each year from 1900 through 1915. The earlier immigrants, who had come predominantly from the British Isles and northern Europe, had participated in the development of a young, growing country. After 1900 the immigrants came increasingly from countries of eastern and southern Europe. Because of their differing customs and traditions, they were looked down upon by the earlier arrivals who considered them only one notch above the Negro on the social scale and invariably relegated them to menial, unskilled tasks. These immigrants were becoming an increasing threat to "purist" Anglo-Saxon Americans, and concern was rising about the pollution of native American stock. They were blamed for many evils of the times, such as increased crime and delinquency, slum conditions, prostitution, poor citizenship, and depression of wages. Unrest grew until the government was forced to do something about limiting immigration. In 1917 a literacy test was made a requirement for admission into the country but was ineffective in controlling immigration. In 1924 the National Origins Act was passed limiting the number of immigrants to 150,000 per year and setting up a quota system based upon the proportion of immigrants from each country who were here in 1920. This act sounded the death knell to immigration.

[7]Smillie, W. *Public Health—Its Promise for the Future.* New York, The Macmillan Company, 1955, Frontispiece.

Education An increasing desire to democ-
ratize and provide free education for all who were able to
profit by it continued to per-
meate the American experience. Public education expanded, and by
1930 nearly all states had passed laws making education compulsory
through age 16. High schools, which had geared their programs
primarily for those preparing for college, were increasingly attended
by students from all walks of life. By 1930 there were 3.5 million
students enrolled in high school.[8] Curricula were no longer meeting
the needs of the majority, and there was agitation for change.
Courses in manual training, home economics, typewriting, agriculture, and vocational education appeared.

Americans are a practical people, and their fundamental instinct
toward preparation for service was strong and instrumental in shaping one of the biggest innovations after 1900—the junior college. This
new kind of program answered the needs of a growing industry and
expanding technology. Business leaders influenced its development.
There were new demands for training at the technical and semiprofessional levels. New occupations, such as engineering assistants and
junior accountants, were opening up, and a new kind of initial preparation was needed. Before the war, with few exceptions, the junior
college was accepted primarily as offering the first 2 years of a 4-year
academic program. After the war there was a trend toward adding
terminal and semiprofessional programs. In 1900 there were eight
private junior colleges each with 100 or more students, and by 1934
there were 521 junior colleges. Of these, 302 were private and 219
public with a total enrollment of 107,807.[9]

Higher education in this part of the twentieth century was marked
by curriculum exploration and experimentation, rapid expansion,
growing student enrollment, and an increasing trend toward coeduca-
tion. Continuing attempts were made to clarify and redefine the aims
and objectives of higher education in American society. There was a
yearning for stability and a necessity for change. During the first 20
years of the new century educational programs were subjected to
serious scrutiny, and repeated attempts were made to develop a

[8]Hackett, L., and Kendrick, B. *The United States Since 1865.* New York, F. S. Crofts and
Company, 1935, p. 691.
[9]Brick, M. *Form and Focus for the Junior College Movement.* New York, Bureau of
Publications, Teachers College, Columbia University, 1964, pp. 24-25.

curriculum more relevant to contemporary society. There was experimentation with curriculum design and methods of teaching. A system of free electives soon gave way to one of group requirements. New breadth of knowledge was included, and general education developed.

Continuous remodeling of the curriculum slackened in the twenties. Universities had reached maturity. State universities had begun their growth toward the gigantic institutions they were to become. A new relationship was developing between the federal government and higher education. The university had accepted its responsibility for the advancement of knowledge and for the preparation of its graduates to meet the needs of the country.

In the twenties the scientific approach had become accepted as basic to progress, and industrialists were beginning, more and more, to realize the value of science in the development of technology. It was about this time that large-scale industrialists, whose products were based on scientific knowledge, set up their own laboratories for industrial research. Thus, they were assured that new and improved products and methods of production would be developed by means of technology.

Graduate programs emphasizing specialization and professional schools expanded and improved. The federal government was turning more and more to institutions of higher learning in meeting national needs. The findings and recommendations of the Flexner Study of Medical Schools, supported by the Rockefeller Foundation in 1910, had a profound effect on the quality of medical education as well as that of other professions.

In contrast to other countries, higher education in America developed without any centralized plan or governmental authority. Thus, it was characterized by the variety of its colleges and universities—public and private, large and small, men's and women's—and also by the diversity of its programs and offerings.

Women's colleges continued to increase in the early part of the century. They still used the model of men's colleges which emphasized classical and scholarly activities. They tended to ignore the needs of the country and the contribution that educated women could make toward meeting these needs. It was during this time that the home economics movement began, stimulated by the passage, in 1914, of the Smith-Lever Act which extended education in agriculture and home economics. The women leaders in this movement were service-oriented rather than reform-oriented and emphasized science rather than the humanities. There were no models available to them such as had been the case in the development of women's colleges. Consequently, institutes, departments, and colleges of home economics appeared in the land-grant colleges whose purpose was to use the knowledge of the laboratory to benefit the people. The home economics programs, similar to those in nursing, were practical and applied, with emphasis on bringing knowledge of sewing and cooking to the people. It was not until after 1920 that the scientific, educational, psychologic, and sociologic principles underlying the practical aspects were considered and that curricula designed to include both theory and practice appeared.

Women's colleges reached their peak about 1920. By this time women accounted for almost half of all college students. As college education became accepted as basic to success for both men and women, the glamour of being an educated woman began to fade and the percentage of women attending college started to decline. After 1930 women increasingly attended coeducational institutions, and no new women's colleges were founded.

Women

After 1900 the role of women continued to expand. The fight for women's suffrage reached gigantic proportions, and many women were personally involved. The Prohibition movement also involved a large number of women, and their efforts had a great deal to do with the enactment by Congress in 1920 of the Volstead Act. This act prohibited the sale, manufacture, or transportation of all intoxicating beverages throughout the country. Through their crusade efforts women became increasingly knowledgeable about the intricacies of the governmental process. After suffrage was granted some used their new knowledge in pursuing political careers.

More and more women worked in the offices of business and industrial firms. The earlier transition from sewing in the home to making garments in the factory was paralleled by the movement from home management to business endeavors. By the beginning of the war women had virtually conquered the stenographic field.

College women were entering many of the professions, and new opportunities were becoming available almost daily. The role of the wife and mother in the family was changing. Some college women

were choosing careers instead of marriage, and there was much discussion about whether women could pursue both marriage and a
career—this controversy is still going on today.

During World War I women were mobilized for the war effort by
the Women's Committee of National Defense set up by President
Wilson. Opportunities were opened up to them on a scale never
before conceived possible. Millions replaced men who had left their
jobs and, as during the Civil War, proved they could do the work
equally as well, if not better. By the end of the war women were
firmly entrenched in many jobs that had previously been open only
to men. The census in 1920 listed 572 occupations; of these, women
were actively engaged in 537.[10] By 1930 one quarter of all women
16 years of age and over were in the labor force.[11]

After the war, with the passage of the Equal Suffrage Act, much
of the militancy of women subsided. They were enjoying the fruits
of the booming economy and their new-found freedom, and the
Flapper era took over. A revolution occurred in women's fashions. A
flat-chested figure and short skirts with long waists became the
approved mode of the day. Women bobbed their hair, smoked
cigarettes, drove cars, invaded speakeasies, and participated in athletics. They flaunted their sexiness and at the same time belittled the
differences between the sexes. There was a whole new relationship
between men and women as they participated together in work and
play. More and more women attended coeducational institutions,
and the decline of women's colleges began.

The Flapper era came to a close by 1930. This era, though short,
gave added impetus to the emancipation of women and dispelled
forever the ideal of the frail, genteel gentlewoman.

Social Consciousness
The period between 1900 and
the First World War saw a tremendous awakening of social
consciousness and is referred
to as the "Age of Reform." There were many reasons for this, such
as the exposure of corruption in big business and in all levels of
government through articles in popular magazines which were read
on a mass basis. Theodore Roosevelt referred to the writers of these

[10]Morris, L. D. *Postscript to Yesterday.* New York, Random House, 1947, p. 50.
[11]Bryson, L., ed. *Facing the Future Risks.* New York, Harper and Brothers, 1953, p. 191.

articles as "muckrakers." There was increasing concern about the need for legislation for the benefit of all. The overall level of education had improved, and people in general were more aware of current conditions and problems. The gap between the rich and the poor was widening, and an upper class, with more leisure, was growing. The first generation of college women wanted to prove the value of higher education for women by doing something to help others who were less fortunate. Most important, perhaps, was the general feeling that society rather than the individual was responsible for the conditions under which people lived; therefore, society had a responsibility to change the conditions. The awakening was a mass movement, and no facet of life escaped the concern of the reformers. Individuals and groups became interested in a cause and then devoted all their energies to that one specific area of interest irrespective of the overall needs of the people. There was no unity or coordination of effort with many gaps and much duplication.

The settlement house was at its heyday during the early part of the period and took the lead in agitating for social action. Settlement workers lived and worked in the slums, attempting in many ways to alleviate the miseries of the people. They took leadership through working on committees, persuading government officials, and organizing protest demonstrations and marches—all in the name of social justice. They concerned themselves with such things as housing, working conditions, hours of work for women, child labor, and health. Their efforts contributed to the assumption of responsibility by the individual states for public health, safety, and morals. Their efforts led directly to the establishment by the federal government in 1912 of the Children's Bureau, with its emphasis on the working conditions of women and children. This was the first social legislation enacted by the federal government.

Others approached reform through interest in special diseases, such as tuberculosis and cancer; specific organs, such as blindness or deafness; special groups, such as children and pregnant women; or special phases, such as safety and planned parenthood. Voluntary organizations concerned with these and many other conditions mushroomed. They pioneered and brought their specific problems to the attention of the people. Many which started at the local and state level became national organizations. The whole voluntary public health nursing movement developed at this time.

Large foundations for specific purposes were established by the wealthy industrialists who had previously made contributions to charity. The Carnegie Foundation, the first, was concerned with the diffusion of knowledge. Others soon followed, such as the Rockefeller Foundation with its concern with the well-being of all mankind, the Commonwealth Fund with its interest in child health projects, and the Rosenwald Foundation for Negro education and medical and hospital services. By 1930 there were some 150 foundations with a combined capitalization of one billion dollars.[12]

The reform period was short-lived and terminated with World War I. Its accomplishments, however, were inestimable. It awakened the federal government to its responsibility for social welfare and demonstrated the pioneering and complementary function of the whole voluntary system within the nation.

After the war there was a marked change in the character of social consciousness in America. Emphasis shifted from attempting to change the social and economic ills of society to helping the individual remedy some of his own maladjustments. The idealism of the reform movement was shattered by the war and its aftermath, and further accentuated by failure of the United States to join the League of Nations. The people were preoccupied with acquiring and enjoying the fruits of a booming economy and rejected restrictions of any kind. Those who criticized existing conditions were thought to be un-American. The rugged individualism and hands-off policy of the government, so characteristic of the eighties and nineties, reappeared. The reluctance of the federal government to take any responsibility for social welfare set the stage for voluntary organizations to flourish.

As voluntary organizations proliferated, the need for financial security, coordination of activities, and equalization of monies became a necessity. The first community chest for this purpose was organized in Cleveland in 1914. By 1931 organized charity was the third largest industry in the United States, and there were almost 400 community chests spending as much as 100 million dollars per year.[13] In spite of this growth there were many gaps in meeting the economic, social, and health needs of the people. These gaps did not become apparent until the depression years.

---

[12] Hackett and Kendrick, *op. cit.*, p. 689.
[13] *Ibid.*, p. 689.

The Depression

So life went on in America during the twenties. Even toward the end of the decade there was an air of optimism and a feeling of prosperity throughout the land. Economists, supposed to have their fingers on the pulse of the nation, were undisturbed. On September 3, 1929, the Dow Jones average of stock market prices made its high record for all times. On November 13 the stock market crashed, and prices reached their lowest point. Allen vividly described its impact:

> The disaster which had taken place may be summed up in a single statistic. In a few short weeks it had blown into thin air *thirty billion dollars*, a sum almost as great as the entire cost to the United States of its participation in the World War, and nearly twice as great as the entire national debt.[14]

As the initial shock of the crash dulled, people faced the realities of a growing depression. The depression of the thirties was without parallel in the history of the country and the world. The entire economy slowed down. Business, construction, farming, mining—all were affected. Incomes decreased and markets contracted. Unemployment rose steadily. In 1931 the banks began to close, adding to the apprehension and misery. Nineteen thirty-two and 1933 were the cruelest years of all: almost one-fourth of the labor force was idle; the streets were less crowded; shops were untenanted; the breadlines were longer; and beggars increasingly apparent. Railroad trains were shorter, and only people who could afford gasoline used their own cars.

The effects of the Depression on the individual varied depending upon his age and station in life. Older people lost their jobs, often permanently. High schools had greater attendance than ever before as students were unable to find work. College graduates who were financially able preferred to go to graduate school rather than to remain idle. Hundreds of thousands of the young people who wanted to get married could not afford to. Those in the upper income brackets took cuts in salaries and either dismissed their servants or allowed them to live in without pay. Many in the middle income

[14] Allen, F. L. *Since Yesterday: The Nineteen-Thirties in America, September 3, 1929-September 3, 1939.* New York, Harper and Brothers, 1940, p. 26.

brackets, thrown out of work by contracting business, were forced to do all sorts of menial and poorly paid jobs in order to feed their families. Many had to go on relief for the first time in their lives. The hardest hit of all were the poor. Numerous writers have vividly described the misery of hundreds of homeless living in tin and tarpaper shacks, the despair of those waiting for hours in breadlines, and the tragedy of men fighting like animals over garbage in the streets. New York City Health Department reported in October 1932 that over one-fifth of the pupils in the public schools were suffering from malnutrition. Hundreds of people went without medical care, and doctors felt themselves lucky when a patient paid a bill.

Relief agencies of all kinds proliferated and tried desperately to meet overwhelming demands. The resources of private organizations were not adequate for this task. People turned more and more to Washington for leadership. Maintenance of general prosperity was not regarded as governmental responsibility. President Hoover was against the government's providing direct relief and injecting itself into business. He saw himself as the watchdog of rugged individualism. As the Depression deepened, so did dissatisfaction with the government and the country in general.

Nursing

Although nursing was an accepted and respectable occupation for women by 1900, it was still a fledgling profession and ill equipped for the turmoil ahead. During the next three decades it became intimately involved in and affected by the whole social upheaval with its reform movement, the First World War, and the Depression. Nursing was sustained, however, by its idealism and humanitarianism. Throughout these difficult times it studied, evaluated, and improved its preparation and performance; developed organizations for more effective functioning; and took definite steps toward the development of educational programs within institutions of higher education for some of its members.

By the turn of the century the demand for nurses was growing. More medical care was being given in hospitals; they were becoming better accepted for the care of the sick and were desperate for personnel. Large, small, special, and general hospitals established training schools for nurses at a phenomenal rate with utter disregard for the educational needs of the pupils. The number of schools grew from 452 in 1900 to 1,755 in 1920.[15] A few of these were good but the great majority unbelievably poor. Pupils were a source of cheap labor for the hospitals. They worked long hours and carried the main responsibility for the care of patients, with little or no supervision. Some pupils became a source of direct income and even profit to the hospitals. They were often sent out, during the early part of their training, to care for private patients in their own homes. Considerable fees were charged for this service. Adelaide Nutting reported in 1912 that:

> Out of the entire 692 hospitals from which statistics were recently received, 248 were found sending out their pupils into families in the community for private nursing, for periods ranging from 2 to 26 weeks, the payment for this service in almost all instances going directly to the hospital.[16]

Many graduates of the poor schools were an embarrassment to nursing at a time when the public was demanding better care. It soon became evident that some legal control was necessary to improve and maintain nursing standards. Groups of nurses in each state began to agitate for legislation to control the education of nurses and the practice of nursing. This was the first real effort of nurses as a group to influence legislation. They soon found out, as had the crusaders for women's suffrage, that they needed to know a great deal more about the legislative process. They persevered, and as a result the first state license law was passed in North Carolina in 1903. By 1913 over twenty states had legislation governing the practice of nursing and the education of nurses.[17]

Amidst the chaotic situation in nursing education was a group who felt strongly that nurses should be educated in universities, similar to other professionals. The majority of colleges and universities, however, still offered classical curricula. Nursing, similar to home economics which developed at about this time, was service-oriented and did not fit into the existing pattern of higher education. The first program for the basic preparation of nurses associated with a univer-

[15] Jamieson, E., Sewall, F., and Gjertson, L. *Trends in Nursing History*, 2nd ed. Philadelphia, W. B. Saunders Company, 1960, p. 416.

[16] Nutting, M. A. *Educational Status of Nursing*. Washington, D.C., U.S. Bureau of Education Bulletin 1912, Government Printing Office, 1912, p. 21.

[17] Stewart, I. *The Education of Nurses*, New York, The Macmillan Company, 1950, p. 140.

sity was inaugurated at the University of Minnesota in 1909. About this time there was also some movement toward hospital schools of nursing affiliating with institutions of higher learning. Several hospital schools had collaborative arrangements with colleges and technical schools for science courses and the use of laboratories for their pupils. College and university courses for graduate nurses were being developed. Teachers College took the lead in this. Pupils were beginning to be referred to as students for the first time. High school graduation was a requirement for entrance to several of the leading schools of nursing, and definite efforts were being made by a few to attract college graduates. Slowly progress was being made. Reform in other areas made it easier to bring about improvements in working conditions and shorter hours of work for both pupil and graduate nurses.

Recruitment of adequate numbers of suitable applicants was becoming increasingly difficult. More and more able women were going to college and paying full tuition for 4 years of education in spite of the fact that education for nursing was generally free and only 2 or 3 years in length. There were all kinds of opportunities for women. Everyone seemed to be clamoring for applicants—for teachers, for doctors, for clerical workers, and others. Recruitment problems were not peculiar to nursing. Nursing's problem, however, was particularly acute because unlike the other professions which had established themselves on an educationally sound basis, nursing was getting more and more entrenched into the apprenticeship system which was inadequate for the needs of the growing profession.

The nursing organizations recognized their responsibility for professional leadership and looked again at their purposes and objectives. In 1911 the Nurses' Associated Alumnae became the American Nurses' Association. By 1912 public health nurses recognized the need for an organization concerned with their particular interests, and the National Organization for Public Health Nursing was started. According to Mary Gardner:

> The object of this organization shall be to stimulate responsibility for the health of the community by establishment and extension of public health nursing; to facilitate efficient cooperation between nurses, physicians, boards of trustees, and other persons interested in public health measures; to develop standards and techniques in public health nursing service; to establish a central bureau for information, reference, and assistance in matters pertaining to such services; and to publish

periodicals or issue bulletins from time to time on the accomplishment of the general purposes of this organization.[18]

The National Organization for Public Health Nursing (also see p. 35) differed from the other two national nursing organizations. One of the differences was that membership was open to public health nurses, public health nursing agencies, and interested citizens. One of its strengths from the beginning was in developing cooperative relationships with other health and social agencies.

The same year the American Society of Superintendents of Training Schools for Nurses became the National League for Nursing Education. It appointed an Education Committee which was specifically concerned with the problems of nursing education and the need for greater standardization and uniformity of the educational programs. *The Standard Curriculum for Nursing Schools*, the first tangible step toward improving nursing education, appeared in 1917, and had real impact at this time. It established the National League for Nursing Education as the authoritative source for information concerning nursing education.

The influence of World War I on nursing was both immediate and far-reaching. It resulted in increasing knowledge and concern on the part of the general public, including many college-trained women, about the whole system of nursing education and its weaknesses. Colleges and universities looked at nursing more seriously as a profession "here to stay." It awakened nurses themselves to the inadequacies of nursing education and laid the groundwork for the studies and changes which followed the war.

Recruitment of nurses for the army and the civilian population had immediate priority. Under the leadership of Adelaide Nutting a National Emergency Committee on Nursing was organized. It soon became the Committee on Nursing of the General Medical Board of the Council of National Defense—a committee established by President Wilson. Adelaide Nutting became the Chairman and Ella Phillips Crandall the secretary of the Committee on Nursing. The plan of this committee for supplying a steady flow of nurses included a well-organized, wide-spread student recruitment program which resulted in increased numbers of students and a Student Nurse Reserve of many thousands. Isabel Stewart relates that:

[18] Gardner, M. S. *Public Health Nursing.* New York, The Macmillan Company, 1916, p. 31.

> The cooperation of public-spirited citizens was also stimulated by the close association of nursing and other groups concerned with national defense. This was true especially of the large and influential Women's Committee under Dr. Anna Howard Shaw of suffrage fame, which with its 12,000 state and local branches took over the chief responsibility for filling the Student Nurse Reserve.[19]

The shortage of nurses in hospitals during the war was eased as the student recruitment program got under way. In addition, many hundreds of women volunteered as aides. These were usually well-educated women who wanted to be of service and knew they were not prepared to be nurses.

In addition to the Committee on Nursing, there were two other committees of the Council of National Defense concerned with nursing—the Subcommittee on Public Health Nurses, with Mary Beard as chairman, and the Subcommittee on Hospitals. The problems of coordination between these subcommittees were complex and difficult. Both Ella Crandall and Mary Beard enlisted the services of the American Red Cross. The demand for public health nurses both at home and abroad was increasing. The Red Cross was asked to establish a special roster of public health nurses who were considered war workers. Their patriotic duty was recognized by the Red Cross which issued a special chevron for them to wear. There was a special need for public health nurses in the areas around the military cantonment areas. Mary Lent was loaned by the National Organization for Public Health Nursing to the United States Public Health Service to cooperate with the local and state agencies and develop a public health nursing program for the cantonment areas. This was the first public health nursing service to be established within the federal government.

A concerted attempt to attract some of the college women into nursing became part of the recruitment program. Letters were sent to all the women's and coeducational colleges in the country, as well as to many graduates, to determine their interest in pursuing nursing as a career. In the summer of 1918 the Vassar Training Camp was set up for college graduates and offered them a preparatory course with the assurance that it would shorten the length of training for nursing. Over 418 attended, and about one-third of these later graduated from schools of nursing and assumed leadership roles in nursing.

[19]Stewart, I., *op cit.*, p. 196.

Currents set in motion by the war continued after the armistice. A better-informed public became increasingly concerned about the health of the people and the supply and preparation of nurses to meet the growing demands of society. Public health nursing services expanded rapidly. As the need for adequate personnel increased, so did questions about the function and preparation of the public health nurse. The Rockefeller Foundation, which had previously given financial assistance to the National Organization for Public Health Nursing, set up a conference for the consideration of some of these questions. In 1918 Dr. C-E. A. Winslow was appointed chairman of the committee to study the whole problem of public health nursing education. It soon became evident that any study of this kind must include nursing and nursing education. The committee was broadened and renamed the Committee for the Study of Nursing Education. Josephine Goldmark was appointed director of the study which extended over a period of 3 years. Some of the recommendations of this study were:

> The quality of applicants and programs of nursing education should be strengthened and improved generally; schools of nursing should work toward increased educational and financial independence; the course should be shortened from three years to twenty-eight months by the elimination of non-educational and repetitive services; subsidiary workers should be prepared and licensed for the care of certain less critically ill patients; emphasis should be placed on special preparation, beyond the basic nursing course, for administrators and teachers for schools òf nursing and for public health nurses; the university schools of nursing should be further developed and strengthened.[20]

There were two important and immediate results of this last recommendation: the founding in 1923 of both the Yale University School of Nursing, financed by the Rockefeller Foundation, and the Frances Payne Bolton School of Nursing at Western Reserve University, financed by Frances Payne Bolton. Miss Bolton was a wealthy and influential citizen who became very much interested in University education for nurses as a result of the Goldmark Report.

The period of the twenties was one of turmoil, reevaluation, and experimentation. Schools of nursing proliferated. Prospective nursing students, recruitment personnel, nurses, and nurse educators wanted and needed more specific and definitive information about the entire nursing situation. In 1925 a program for grading schools of nursing

[20] Roberts, M. *American Nursing*, New York, The Macmillan Company, 1954, p. 179.

was approved by the three national nursing organizations, and a year later the Committee on the Grading of Nursing Schools came into being. It was composed of 21 members—14 of whom represented national organizations interested in the quality and availability of nursing. The Committee undertook three major projects: a study of the supply and demand for nursing service, a job analysis of nurses, and the grading of nursing schools. Grading of schools was accomplished in 1929 and repeated in 1932. As a result several hundred of the poorer schools closed their doors, and many others improved their educational programs.

Although early connections between schools of nursing and institutions of higher education were sporadic and without uniformity, they continued to multiply. By 1931 there were 67 schools of nursing with some kind of college or university relationship, 12 percent of these being affiliated with junior colleges.[21] At the same time college education for graduate nurses was becoming more available. These developments in nursing education brought with them a whole new set of perplexing problems relating to organization, administration, financing, curriculum, and faculty and student qualifications. A series of conferences was held to discuss these problems, and there was a consensus that the advantages in these new relationships outweighed the disadvantages. The Committees on University Schools of the National League for Nursing Education took the leadership in these deliberations and continued to study the situation. In 1933 the Association of Collegiate Schools of Nursing was formed with the following purposes:

> To develop nursing education on a professional and collegiate level, to promote and strengthen relationships between schools of nursing and institutions of higher education, and to promote a study and experimentation in nursing service and nursing education.[22]

Most of the energies of the leaders in nursing during the period following the war were directed toward studying and improving the educational preparation of nurses. A few postgraduate courses were becoming available in colleges and universities for the preparation of head nurses. Graduate nurses were assuming head nurse positions in hospitals. Postgraduate courses were also available for the prepara-

---

[21] *Proceedings of the 37th Annual Convention of the National League for Nursing Education in 1931*, p. 134.
[22] Stewart, *op. cit.*, p. 231.

tion of teachers, supervisors, and administrators in nursing. Some hospitals were developing courses for nurses who wished further clinical knowledge in special areas such as pediatrics, maternity, and the operating room. With the exception of public health nursing, universities did not accept any responsibility for the preparation of nurses for the practice of nursing. The first grading study showed that even at the very height of national prosperity many private duty nurses were unemployed. There were far more nurses than could be employed under existing conditions. On the other hand, there were too few nurses qualified for positions demanding special knowledge and skills.

By the end of the twenties the deepening depression was affecting all aspects of the American economy, and unemployment among graduate nurses was becoming pronounced. They did not escape the weary round of job hunting, reduced salaries, depleted savings, or even the bread lines. Many of the hospitals which had discontinued their schools of nursing employed graduate nurses for the first time. The numbers employed increased with the severity of the depression, Many graduates were willing to work for low salaries and even to give free service in exchange for room and board. The outcome of this was positive. Hospital administrators realized that graduate nurses gave better care to patients than did students, and a whole new area of service opened up for graduate nurses. New possibilities for the development of more independence for schools of nursing loomed on the horizon.

Nursing withstood the stresses and strains of the first three decades of the twentieth century and matured in the process. Recognition of the necessity for better education for nurses resulted in considerable improvement in nursing programs within hospitals. In addition, the foundation for future developments in collegiate education for nurses was firmly laid.

Public Health Nursing

Public health nursing really came into its own during the first three decades of the twentieth century. It clarified its purposes, preparation, and organization. By 1900 the germ theory of the cause of disease was well established. Public health endeavors for the most part were geared toward the application of this theory in the control and prevention of communicable disease, with major emphasis placed upon control of the environment. In spite of these efforts the incidence of communicable disease was widespread. Williams[23] has reported that between 1890 and 1910 there was more than three times the number of deaths from typhoid fever in the United States than in some of the other countries of the world. The philosophy that the government should be responsible for the health of the community had not as yet permeated the state and local health departments. The federal government was beginning to show a little interest in its responsibility for public health, and the need for more adequate statistics about people as a whole was beginning to be recognized. The Census Bureau was established in 1902 and the Death Registration Area in 1900. In 1902 Congress also passed an act which gave legal authority for the first time to the Surgeon General of the United States Public Health Service to hold periodic conferences with the State and Territorial Health Officers in order to promote the interest of public health.

Many of the people involved in the reform movement were concerned about the poor health situation and the need for legislation to improve the health of the people. Industrial and technologic developments had stimulated the economy of the country, and the accumulated wealth provided a means of support for community health. Voluntary health agencies concerned with a particular disease or condition proliferated. The rapid growth of these agencies was due in part to the constant threat of communicable disease, the ineffectiveness of health departments in alleviating this threat, and the widespread feeling of social consciousness with its urgency to improve the plight of the poor. The philosophy underlying the development of voluntary health agencies was that of the importance of community action in the protection of the health of the individual. This was exemplified by the interest and involvement of citizens in establishing and financing the services that were provided.

As the services offered by the voluntary health agencies expanded, so did the demand for nurses in specialized programs. The tuberculosis crusade was the first to recognize the contribution of the nurse as a teacher of hygiene and sanitation in the control of tuberculosis.

[23] Williams, R. C. *The United States Public Health Service.* Bethesda, Maryland, The Commissioned Officers Association of the United States Public Health Service, Box 5874, 1951, p. 140.

The high mortality rate of infants led to the development of infant welfare stations, and more nurses were demanded to work in this specialized area. It was not long before nurses were being sought to function in specialized areas such as communicable disease, tuberculosis, venereal disease, mental health, schools, factories, and many others.

The voluntary movement in district nursing, which mushroomed after the turn of the century, was consistent with the development of other voluntary health agencies. The citizens recognized the needs for nursing care to sick people in their homes and in turn organized and contributed funds to meet these needs. The voluntary nursing agencies contributed by innovating new programs, demonstrating the need for public health nursing, and supplementing governmental nursing services. This was exemplified by Lillian Wald at Henry Street when she demonstrated the value of a nurse in the public schools. As a result of this experiment, the Board of Education in New York City, in 1902, employed the first school nurse in the United States. There were several leaders in nursing who thought that public health nursing should be a responsibility of government; some local health departments were employing nurses.

Public health nursing was well established by the time the reform movement in public health took place around 1910. Although the general reform movement was beginning to show some signs of waning by this time, it resulted in legislation and philosophic changes in society which strongly influenced the whole development and approach of public health. It resulted in health legislation which gave authority to the states for the protection of the individual and made the health of the individual a community responsibility. At the same time the emphasis in the control of disease was broadening to include the promotion of the health of the individual in his environment, rather than just controlling the environment. It was at this time that district nursing, which had pioneered in health promotion and disease prevention by working with people in their own homes, became a ready and able partner in the whole public health movement. According to Winslow public health nurses provided the first effective link between a planned community health program and the individual family in the home. Winslow further states that "for what the nursing profession has accomplished and for the leadership of the board member group in that accomplishment, we owe an incalculable debt of gratitude."[24] It was at this time that the functions of the district nurse expanded and more nearly met those of a public health nurse, as envisioned by Lillian Wald when she started district nursing services at Henry Street.

Public health nursing services were organized in a variety of ways. They were offered by large and small visiting nurse associations, medical dispensaries, and boards of health. In some instances visiting nurse associations in the larger cities sold services to smaller surrounding communities or combined their services with boards of health or boards of education. In 1909 the Metropolitan Life Insurance Company, as a result of an experiment with Henry Street, offered nursing service to certain of its policy holders. Its plan was to affiliate with existing agencies rather than to duplicate services, and to employ its own nurses only when no other service was available. By 1928 it had affiliations with 953 organizations and employed an independent staff of 592 nurses. There was also great variation in the development of rural public health nursing services, depending on the needs and resources of individual communities. Public health nurses could be found working under many auspices—including the Red Cross.

Irrespective of the kind of arrangement, stress was laid upon organizing to meet the needs of the community, and upon the premise that each local community must determine how its service should be organized. In spite of the flexibility and diversity of the programs and agencies, some principles of administration in public health nursing were evolving. Some of these were: the need for sound financing of public health nursing; the necessity for the involvement of community people in establishing and financing the program; the recognition that the program of the agency should be based upon the needs of the community; the necessity for nursing to collaborate with other health and social agencies in the community in order to avoid gaps and duplication in service; and the importance of records and statistics as necessary tools in the development of public health nursing. At the same time the relationship of the health of the family to the health of the community was beginning to be recognized, and the family as a whole was becoming the focus for the public health nurse.

[24]Winslow, C-E. A. Housing and health. *The Public Health Nurse,* 32:437, July 1940.

As the role and activities of the district nurse broadened and diversified, it soon became apparent that further educational preparation beyond the hospital was necessary. A few of the visiting nurse associations instituted in-service education programs for their nurses, but there were no organized programs for the preparation of district nurses. The first course for graduate nurses who wished to specialize in district nursing was established by the Instructive District Nursing Association of Boston in 1906. The course was 4 months in length and included lectures and practice. Several of the larger visiting nurse associations established similar courses in an attempt to meet the need for better-prepared district nurses. It was not until 1910, when a Department of Nursing and Health for graduate nurses was established at Teachers College, Columbia University, that institutions of higher learning assumed any responsibility for the education of public health nurses. The Department of Nursing and Health was an outgrowth of a course in Hospital Economics for graduate nurses established at Teachers College in 1899 and sponsored by the Society of Superintendents of Training Schools. The course had been designed to prepare women for administrative and teaching positions in hospitals but had never been satisfactorily developed because of lack of funds. A gift of $150,000 from Helen Jenkins made the Department of Nursing and Health financially stable and permanent. This was the first time that money was given to support any nursing education in the United States. Three programs of study were offered: the preparation of teachers and supervisors for training schools; the preparation of administrators of hospitals and training schools; and the preparation of public health nurses.[25]

As a result of the program at Teachers College, some of the visiting nurse associations which offered special public health nursing courses for the preparation of their own staff developed collaborative relationships with colleges and universities. For example, the course at the Cleveland Visiting Nurse association was transferred to Western Reserve University in 1911, and the one conducted by the Instructive District Nursing Association of Boston was transferred to Simmons College in 1912. By 1921 there were 15 colleges and universities offering courses in public health nursing which met the educational standards developed by the National Organization for Public Health Nursing.[26] By 1929 the National Organization for

[25] Nutting, *op. cit.*, pp. 8-9.
[26] Strong, A. The education of public health nurses. *The Public Health Nurse*, 13:226, May 1921.

Public Health Nursing had established a procedure for grading post-graduate courses in public health nursing, and had approved courses that met the following minimum requirements: a qualified nurse director; affiliation with a school of collegiate grade; a budget; and an academic-year program with didactic and field instruction. By this time, partly as a result of the introduction into universities of public health nursing courses, 5-year undergraduate programs in nursing were established in a few colleges and universities. Seven of the approved postgraduate public health nursing courses were connected with 5-year university programs and provided the fifth year in public health nursing to an increasing number of undergraduate nursing students.[27]

It was during the twenties that public health recognized the relationship of the health of the individual to the economic security of the community and assumed responsibility for community health. By 1920 all the states and most of the large cities had health departments which were staffed by large numbers of people. The largest proportion of professional workers were public health nurses. The importance of health education, both on an individual and a broad community-wide basis, had its beginnings during this time and was fostered by the developments in mass communication, such as the radio, moving pictures, and the increasing circulation of newspapers and magazines. In 1924 the Shephard-Towner Act was passed which gave money to the states on a matching basis to enable each state to establish a program for the promotion of the welfare and hygiene of mothers and infants. This act, which was vigorously opposed by many as a violation of states' rights, established the pattern to be followed later by the federal government, that of awarding monies on a matching basis to the states for the alleviation of a variety of health hazards.

Paralleling developments in public health were developments in public health nursing. Public health nursing was in its heyday during the twenties. It was the standard bearer for both the improvement and expansion of health services. It took leadership in establishing standards of nursing practice; demanded academic education for public health nurses; worked with citizens and other professionals in developing and improving services; and established a sound basis for cost and time studies. It collaborated with other professional organi-

[27]National Organization for Public Health Nursing. Post graduate courses in public health nursing. *The Public Health Nurse*, 21:94, February 1929.

zations in carrying out the first real census of public health nurses, which became a model for later studies. Public health nursing became part of both state and local health departments and expanded its services in both rural and urban areas. It influenced and was in turn influenced by health and welfare legislation.

Public health nurses brought health services directly to the people and were welcomed into the homes of the rich and poor alike. They not only gave bedside nursing care but also interpreted the latest knowledge of disease prevention and health promotion. They helped to broaden the nation's concept of health. They also demonstrated that prevention of disease and promotion of health, as well as care of the sick, were a responsibility of nursing.

The family had become recognized as the unit of service for the public health nurse. At the same time, in spite of this, many agencies were employing specialists in such areas as venereal disease, tuberculosis, maternal and child health, and school nursing. There was growing recognition that specialists were needed for leadership, but also that duplication and gaps in service resulted. By the middle of the twenties the trend was toward generalization of services, through which one staff nurse, adequately supervised and supported by well-trained supervisors and consultants, gave total service to an individual family.

The first census of public health nurses in the United States as of January 1, 1924, carried out by the National Organization for Public Health Nursing, was remarkable in its organization and management. The cooperation of those participating was a real tribute to the National Organization for Public Health Nursing. It was the most comprehensive study of its kind to date and included 752 cities of populations over 10,000 as well as smaller cities and rural areas of the country. This first official census showed that there were 3,267 organizations employing 11,152 full-time graduate nurses.[28] It also revealed variation in financing, and gaps and duplication of services. Forty-seven percent of agencies were supported wholly by public funds; an additional 28 percent received some public funds; and 25 percent were supported wholly by private funds. Nursing service was

[28] National Organization for Public Health Nursing. Census of public health nurses in the United States, January 1, 1924. *The Public Health Nurse*, 18:24-27, January 1926.

entirely free in all but 24 percent of the agencies.[29]

One of the statistical problems encountered by the National Organization for Public Health Nursing in planning the census had been the lack of an actual definition of public health nursing. As a result, information about qualifications had not been included in the census. A year later, the American Public Health Association, National Organization for Public Health Nursing, and State and Provincial Health authorities formed a joint committee to consider minimal qualifications for public health nursing at the staff, supervisory, and director levels. They recommended qualifications for 1925 and projected them for 1930. It is interesting to note that two years of high school was acceptable in 1925 for all three levels, but completion of high school was a requirement by 1930. Professional, academic, and experience requirements were progressive, and the 1930 qualifications for staff nurses included theoretic and practical experience in one or more of the following: public health nursing, communicable disease nursing, tuberculosis nursing, hospital social services, or mental hygiene. Qualification for supervisors and directors required at least 2 years of public health nursing experience and a recognized public health nursing course, including theory and practice in an education institution. College education, or at least 2 years beyond the minimal educational requirements, was considered desirable.

The next few years were tremendously important ones for public health nursing. A manual presenting general underlying principles and guidelines for public health nursing was published in 1926, and revised in 1932. The first cost studies for public health nursing were published in 1926, and increasing numbers of comparative cost figures became available for use in planning. An appraisal form was developed 2 years later and was instrumental in directing attention to both quality and quantity of service.

By the early thirties the effects of the Depression were omnipresent. Public health nursing services had to be curtailed. Salaries decreased. Unemployment was on the rise. However, public health nursing was, on the whole, in a peculiarly fortunate position to withstand the Depression. It had formulated its objectives and worked out

[29]Clark, M. The census and public health nursing traditions. *The Public Health Nurse* 18:464, 465, 467, August 1926.

a sound basis of organization. As the need for service increased, public health nursing was in a position to respond and to become more intimately involved with the community in meeting these needs.

Summary The period between 1900 and the New Deal was bisected by the First World War with all its horror, and ended with the greatest depression the country had ever known—a depression which resulted in the New Deal and a change in the whole relationship between rugged individualism and the role of the government. The challenges to previously accepted ideas and beliefs were forceful and insistent. Endemic values were changing and priorities being reordered. There was now a general feeling that:

> The doors should no longer be wide open to immigrants. They were a growing threat to Anglo-Saxonism and were held responsible by many for a large share of the ills of society.
>
> Society and not the individual was responsible for poverty, and society must do something about these social ills. The need for social reform was given high priority.
>
> The gap between the rich and the poor was widening. The rich must organize and contribute to help the poor.
>
> Education was not just important for a free society, but was necessary for a democracy if it were to survive.
>
> Americans were a practical people, and their education should be practical and relevant.
>
> Higher education was equally as valuable for women as men.
>
> The suburbs were increasingly desirable places for middle- and upper-class families to live and raise their children.
>
> Women should have equal rights but until this became reality should demand them.
>
> Science, technology, and research were basic to industry, education, and progress itself.
>
> There was more than one cause for environmental and disease conditions.
>
> The size and composition of the American family was changing.
>
> An overriding optimism prevailed, even right up to the time of the Depression.

The effects of war on any country are profound and incalculable. The aftermath of World War I was no exception. The prewar frenzy for social, legislative, and educational reform died out after the war. Emphasis shifted from helping others to that of enjoying the good things of life—many of which had been made possible by progress in transportation, industry, and education.

The Depression tested individual and voluntary effort to solve the problems of the country almost to the breaking point. The resources of private individuals and groups, no matter how dedicated, were just not adequate for the task. The results of the Depression demanded that the federal government assume a whole new kind of responsibility for the general welfare. A new partnership between the government and voluntary organizations began to develop, and there was a growing realization that:

> Although individualism was still important, it might have to be submerged for the good of all the people.
>
> The government not only should but must assume responsibility for the general welfare.

The idealism and humanitarianism which continued to dominate nursing during this period hampered reform in both the education and practice of nursing. Society idealized the nurse as an "angel of mercy" who soothed the feverish brows of the sick. Thus, persons who selected nursing as a career were conditioned by society's views and tended to perpetuate them. This image, with its implications for dedicated service, was to haunt nursing for many years and put a damper on the reforms necessary for the development of nursing as a scholarly profession.

At the same time, changes were occurring in society at large which pinpointed the need for better education for nurses. It was generally accepted that education was necessary for a society's survival, and public education became more readily available for everyone. Higher education became acceptable for women, and the idea that women could pursue both a career and marriage gained momentum. Graduate education expanded, professional schools developed, and research became important for progress.

Nursing was struggling to get into the main stream of education, but was having a difficult time because of an entrenched apprenticeship system which it could not shake, despite valiant efforts by a few dedicated individuals. Also, for much of the period curricula in colleges were still oriented toward the classics, and this made it doubly difficult to conceive of nursing, which was practice-oriented, as being included in the existing structure of higher education. Other professions for women were developing, such as social work and home economics, and were faced with a similar dilemma. However, as these professions developed, men also became attracted to them. In many instances it was men who took the leadership in establishing standards for education, which were then equally applicable to the men and women in the profession. Nursing, on the other hand, was exclusively a female occupation and was under the domination of physicians. The physicians assumed leadership over the educational standards for nurses as well as those for the medical profession. Thus, the educational standards were higher for the physician, who was usually a man, and lower for the nurse, who was usually a woman. Perhaps if men had been attracted to nursing in its formative stage, the father image of the physician would not have become so strongly entrenched, and nursing would have moved more quickly into the mainstream of higher education.

The unchecked growth of hospital training schools for nurses and the lack of uniform standards for practice and education were an overriding concern of nursing during this period. Some of the thoughtful leaders in nursing realized that nursing had to get itself organized and set up its own standards if it were to develop and survive as a profession.

At the beginning of the century when the reform movement reached its zenith, there was feverish activity in all areas with no coordination of efforts or any overall master plan. It was almost as if there was a sudden reawakening of the need for reform in every area of life. The important thing was to bring about change, and it really did not matter too much who selected which endeavor. Individualism was the order of the day, and there was ample opportunity for individuals or groups to develop their special interests without government interference. Thus, it was natural for special interest groups in nursing to evolve, and the stage was set for the development of public health nursing as a separate entity.

Reform in nursing took place within the context of where nursing was practiced. Institutional nursing was greatly influenced by the hospital with its boundaries and problems, whereas public health nursing, which was practiced outside of the hospital, was more closely related to the community and the forces affecting society as a whole. With the increase in scientific knowledge and technology the hospital became more acceptable for the care of the sick, and the focus of nursing, as well as of medicine, was centered on the sick individual. Nurses needed knowledge about disease and its treatment in order to carry out the medical plan of care. Students were the primary providers of nursing care in the hospital and were ideal handmaidens to the physician. Public health nurses, on the other hand, were translating the benefits of scientific knowledge directly to the family in the home for the purpose of health promotion and disease prevention. Trained nurses were the primary providers of nursing care and were not necessarily dependent upon a medical plan of care. Team relationships with the physician and other health professionals were developing as it became more and more evident that the health needs of families could not be met by any one discipline working in isolation. The beginnings of the public health team consisting of the public health physician, the public health nurse, and the sanitarian were gaining impetus.

Tremendous energy was expended on defining educational standards for nurses, both by institutional nursing and public health nursing. The major thrust was toward establishing uniform standards for nursing education and practice. Institutional nursing recognized the need for preparing administrators and teachers in institutions of higher learning, and a few programs one year in length were established. Public health nursing at the same time was giving high priority to the need for better-educated nurses in order to provide better service to patients. One-year university programs were established with public health nursing practice as the objective. Educational standards were developed for staff nurses, supervisors, and administrators in public health nursing and were included as part of the requirements for employment under many of the Civil Service Commissions. Also, in-service education, in which the employing agency took responsibility for conducting educational programs to help nurses keep abreast of new developments in order to bring this knowledge to their patients, was reinforced. The public health nurse was becoming a familiar and welcome figure in the homes of people in all walks of life. Developments in transportation, particularly the Model-T Ford, made it possible for her to reach more people and to extend her services to rural areas. She was often the only person in smaller communities who was concerned about the health status, and in many instances her endeavors led to the development of full-time health departments.

The rapid development of voluntary visiting nurse associations with strong citizen involvement speeded the development of sound personnel policies and regular working hours for public health nurses. Citizen participation in public health nursing culminated in the establishment of the National Organization for Public Health Nursing with its emphasis on lay membership. The importance of working collaboratively with other professionals in solving health problems early became one of the armamentaria of public health nurses, and its importance was vividly demonstrated in 1923 when Public Health Nursing became a section in the American Public Health Association.

Nursing research did not take on stature until a much later time, but a research approach, the value of statistics, fact-finding, and the ordering of data were early tools of public health nursing. Time and cost studies in public health nursing were models that were used by other groups in studying costs. Collaborative relationships with other national organizations in the census of public health nurses also became a model for multidiscipline collaboration.

Public health nursing was in its heyday during this period. No endeavor was too great, and every aspect of the life of the family and the community was the territory of the public health nurse. The independent functions of nursing were demonstrated, although not identified, and a vision of nursing as a profession was created.

REFERENCES

Allen, F. L. The Big Change. New York, Harper and Brothers, 1952.
_____ Since Yesterday: The Nineteen-Thirties in America, September 3, 1929-September 3, 1939. New York, Harper and Brothers, 1940.
Berelson, B. Graduate Education in the United States. New York, McGraw-Hill Company, 1960.
Brick, M. Form and Focus for the Junior College Movement. New York, Bureau of Publications, Teachers College, Columbia University, 1964.
Bryson, L., ed. Facing the Future Risks. New York, Harper and Brothers, 1953.
Clark, M. The census and public health nursing traditions. The Public Health Nurse, 18:464-467, August 1926.
Committee on the Grading of Nursing Schools. Nursing Schools Today and Tomorrow. New York City, 1934.
Deming, D. Milestones of the past fifteen years in public health nursing. Amer. J. Public Health, 29:128-134, February 1939.
DeVane, W. C. Higher Education in Twentieth Century America. Cambridge, Mass., Harvard University Press, 1965.
Dowd, D. Modern Economic Problems in Historical Perspective. Boston, D. C. Heath and Company, 1962.
Dulles, F. The United States Since 1865. Ann Arbor, The University of Michigan Press, 1959.

Gardner, M. S. Public Health Nursing. New York, The Macmillan Company, 1916.

Hackett, L., and Kendrick, B. The United States Since 1865. New York, F. S. Crofts and Company, 1935.

Jamieson, E., Sewall, F., and Gjertson, L. Trends in Nursing History, 2nd ed. Philadelphia, W. B. Saunders and Company, 1960.

Morris, L. D. Not So Long Ago. New York, Random House, 1949.

─────── Postscript to Yesterday. New York, Random House, 1947.

Mowry, F. The Urban Nation 1920-1960. New York, Hill and Wang, 1965.

National Organization for Public Health Nursing. Census of public health nurses in the United States—1924. The Public Health Nurse, 18:24-27, January 1926.

─────── Census of public health nurses in the United States, January 1, 1924. The Public Health Nurse, 18:249-313, June 1926.

─────── Post graduate courses in public health nursing. The Public Health Nurse, 21:93-95, February 1929.

─────── Principles and Practices in Public Health Nursing Including Cost Analysis. New York, The Macmillan Company, 1932.

─────── Standardizing qualifications for public health nursing positions. The Public Health Nurse, 17:297-299, June 1925.

Newcomer, M. A Century of Higher Education for American Women. New York, Harper and Brothers, 1959.

Nutting, M. A. Educational Status of Nursing. Washington, U. S. Bureau of Education Bulletin 1912, Government Printing Office, 1912.

Petry, L. Basic professional curricula in nursing leading to degrees. Amer. J. Nurs., 37:287-297, March 1937.

Proceedings of the 37th Annual Convention of the National League for Nursing Education in 1931, p. 134.

Rae, J. B. The American Automobile. Chicago, University of Chicago Press, 1965.

Roberts, M. American Nursing. New York, The Macmillan Company, 1954.

Schlesinger, A. Age of Roosevelt—Crisis of the Old Order 1919-1933. Boston, Houghton Mifflin Company, 1957.

Smillie, W. Public Health—Its Promise for the Future. New York, The Macmillan Company, 1955.

Stewart, I. The Education of Nurses. New York, The Macmillan Company, 1950.

Strong, A. The education of public health nurses. The Public Health Nurse, 13:226-230, May 1921.

Williams, R. C. The United States Public Health Service. Bethesda, Maryland, The Commissioned Officers Association of the United States Public Health Service, Box 5874, 1951.

Winslow C-E. A. Housing and health. The Public Health Nurse, 32:434-439, July 1940.

CHAPTER 3

The Period From the New Deal Through the Johnson Era

The New Deal grew out of a shattering depression and brought with it a myriad of programs of relief, recovery, and reform designed to revitalize the machinery of a troubled nation. It resulted in a new role for the federal government—that of responsible overseer of the general welfare—and added a new dimension to social policy. It also resulted in more willingness on the part of the people to invest in common security at the expense of individual freedom.

The federal government demonstrated its real concern for the growing problems of the country. Between 1935 and the late sixties there was an increasing flow of legislation aimed at improvement of health and welfare, housing and urban development, antidiscrimination in civil rights, fair practices in employment, school desegregation, and aid to education, including nursing education. Ideas generated by the slogans "The New Frontier" of the Kennedy era and

"The Great Society" of the subsequent Johnson era expressed the desire on the part of both the people and the government for an added dimension to the quality of life, and an expansion of opportunity and equality to all facets of society. Achievement of many of these ideas was overshadowed by a widening concern and disillusionment with America's deeper and deeper involvement in the undeclared war in Vietnam. By the end of the period the need for national goals and priorities, and the importance of planning as a means to meet these goals were beginning to come into national focus. Blueprints for such plans as new towns, coordinated transportation systems, programs for control of the environment, and restructured health and welfare systems were on the drawing boards.

Also, by the late sixties the country was well on its way to becoming an urban industrial society. Increases in population, transportation, and industrialization brought with them a whole new set of health and health-related problems. Some of these, such as environmental hazards, crime and delinquency, and drug addiction and its related problems, were a result of the shifting concentration of people. Nurses, along with other health professionals and consumers, were deeply involved in the problems and struggled to reevaluate and redefine their role and purposes to meet these new challenges. Nursing was firmly convinced that it must become truly professional, as only in this way could it integrate and utilize the results of rapid and expanding scientific, technologic, and sociologic knowledge and with others meet the changing health needs of an impatient, better-educated, health-conscious people.

Nursing also believed increasingly in the value of higher education for nurses in contemporary society. By the late sixties it had set its sights in this direction and accepted baccalaureate education as beginning preparation for professional nursing, and graduate education as the base for the preparation of nurse specialists and leaders. Research and writing were gaining acceptance as important professional attributes. Nursing, along with other professions, was caught up in the universal struggle to make its education more relevant.

Nurses, and particularly public health nurses, were participating with an expanding number of community health workers involved in planning and carrying out a complex of new and comprehensive health programs, both voluntary and governmental. As the pattern of health organization was changing, so was the role of nursing and public health nursing. The road ahead was exciting and challenging but far from clear.

Transportation

Transportation, which played so important a role in the early frontiers, was still a dominant factor in the increasing expansion of the country. By the beginning of World War II, the automobile had become a pivot around which much of the life of the people revolved. Production of automobiles came to a standstill during the war as many of the large automobile plants harnessed their machinery and men to produce ships and airplanes. After the war, however, production was resumed. In addition, advances in the design and construction of highways played a big part in the expansion of the automobile. By 1960 four-fifths of all American families owned at least one car and used it mainly for pleasure.[1]

The vast expansion of the automobile had both its good and bad effects, but there is no question about its impact on all aspects of life. The development of the cities, with the flight of the more affluent to the suburbs, could not have happened without the automobile. Parking problems, traffic congestion, violent deaths by accidents, noise, smog, and air pollution increased as the number of automobiles grew. The need for a vast network of more and better highways resulted in the bisection and dissection of farms and villages across the country by thousands of miles of superhighways. In spite of the number of highways, the production of cars outstripped road building, and traffic congestion magnified. As people moved to the suburbs, large shopping centers developed with ample parking facilities. At the same time, because of lack of parking facilities, many of the well-established stores in the center of cities either moved to the suburban shopping centers or were forced to close their doors. Industry began to move out of the central cities as more and more people commuted to work by automobile and as industry became less dependent upon the railroads for transportation of goods and materials.

Americans were on the move with mobility the way of life. Gone were the days when a child was born, lived out his lifespan, and died in the same community. Goods and produce were accessible to everyone, even in some of the remotest parts of the country. At the

[1] Rae, J. B. *The American Automobile.* Chicago, University of Chicago Press, 1965, p. 192.

same time television, radio, and other mass media were constantly reminding the people of the things they could have or that others had. New industries and occupations developed to keep the transportation system operating and to meet the needs of the people for recreational activities made possible by developments in transportation.

The airplane was still in its infancy at the outbreak of hostilities, but the needs of the Second World War hastened its development. After the war commercial airlines expanded, jet planes which could transport large numbers of people around the world in a matter of hours became commonplace, and travel to the moon was a reality. Airports were developed in or adjacent to all the major cities. By the late sixties air congestion had become a serious problem, and the need for more and larger airports to accommodate the superjets and their increased number of passengers was a source of concern. With the increased speed of transportation more stringent methods of disease surveillance became necessary because of the rapidity with which disease could spread from one part of the world to another. The noise-abatement program to reduce the sound of airplanes became a major occupation. Controversy over the supersonic planes was beginning.

In the expansion of transportation there was a partnership between the federal government and private enterprise, with each dependent upon the other. The federal government subsidized highway construction over which the automobile, developed by private enterprise, traveled. Government weather forecasts and air traffic control were necessary for commercial airlines to operate. National and international regulations to control the spread of disease made it possible for airplanes to carry people to all corners of the world. Federal subsidy of railroads made it possible for the railroads to survive during the period of declining traffic. Government expenditures and controls made possible the voluntary coordination of the industrialists to develop the means to meet the needs of the people for transportation.

Industrialization and Technology

During the depression years industrial expansion was practically nil, and many industries cut back production to a minimum. Unemployment soared, and the plight of the workers was desperate. Labor unions, which had been struggling unsuccessfully to organize workers on a nation-wide basis, were able to flourish in this climate. Legislation favorable to the development of strong labor unions was enacted, and the organization of workers in their own behalf was sanctioned by the nation for the first time.

By the beginning of the war, production of goods had resumed, industry was on its way to recovery, and crippling strikes by labor unions were a threat to be reckoned with. Production of domestic goods came to a halt at the outbreak of the war, with the entire industrial and technologic power geared to the war effort. A moratorium on strikes was declared by the labor unions and was one of the factors which contributed to the enormous industrial and technologic growth during the war years. The government and universities collaborated in joint ventures for the development of scientific research and technology to meet the tremendous needs of modern warfare. Once again the American genius for know-how and the practical ingenuity of the people came to the fore. Automobile factories became airplane factories, ships were built at a phenomenal rate, increases in agriculture revolutionized farming, synthetic rubber was developed, new drugs such as penicillin appeared almost daily, strides were made in the treatment of the sick and wounded, and radar was developed and used extensively. The race for atomic weapons was won by the United States, and the war came to an end when atom bombs were dropped on Hiroshima and Nagasaki. The atom bomb ushered in the nuclear age, and a world-wide contest began for supremacy in the development of greater and more devastating war weapons. This contest was destined to change the power structure of the world.

After the war the economy shifted to the production of consumer goods. People who had "done without" for so many years clamored for all sorts of products. The supply at first was small, and inflation was an ever-present threat. The no-strike policy of the labor unions ended, and devastating strikes crippled most of the major industries. In 1947 Congress passed the Taft-Hartley Act in an effort to dilute some of the power of organized labor. There was much opposition to this legislation by the labor unions, and the controversy is still going on today.

The development and expansion of television after the war was probably more important to the country than the expansion of the radio had been after World War I. Dulles[2] estimates that in 1958

[2] Dulles, F. *The United States Since 1865.* Ann Arbor, University of Michigan Press, 1959, p. 514.

there were 50,000,000 television sets in use. Television was bringing into the living room every type of entertainment and spectator sport, political contests, educational programs, war, and commercials. No facet of life was immune. For the first time people were seeing what they were missing, and their desires and aspirations were changed. The distance between the rich and the poor became more visible. At the same time the American people enjoyed a higher standard of living than the world had ever known. Mass distribution of goods was as important as mass production. People in all walks of life were buying and using the same commodities, were seeing the same kind of shows, were reading the same kinds of books, were riding in the same kinds of automobiles, and were traveling to the same places. The differences were in the degree to which people participated, rather than participation only by an elite group.

Scientific and technologic discoveries, which in peace time might have taken many years, advanced at a phenomenal rate during World War II and helped to trigger a whole new concern over environmental health. Development of nerve gas, development and use of DDT and other pesticides and important biologic research such as that in oceanography had unexpected and frightening results. For example, in the fifties scientists began to uncover disturbing facts about DDT's effects on the chain of life—its tendency to accumulate in the fatty tissue of the wild life. Questions were raised about the effect of pesticides even deadlier than DDT in regard to sporadically reported fish kills. The relationship of all of this to human life was disturbingly unclear.

Also in the fifties, Sweden reported high death rates among birds which had eaten methylmercury-coated seeds. Mysteriously fatal "epidemics" among humans were tracked down to methylmercury-coated seeds in Iraq in 1956, in West Pakistan in 1961, and in Guatemela in 1963.[3]

Rachael Carson's book *Silent Spring* was published in 1962. It has been likened to Harriet Beecher Stowe's *Uncle Tom's Cabin* as regards the impact of a literary work upon a great social debate. Robert Rudd, a noted biologist, said of the book:

> *Silent Spring* is biological warning, social commentary and moral reminder. Insistently she calls upon technological man to pause and take stock.[4]

[3]Montague, P., and Montague, C. Mercury: How much are we eating? *Saturday Review*, February 6, 1971, p. 51.
[4]Graham, F. *Since Silent Spring*. Greenwich, Connecticut, Fawcett Publications, Inc., 1970, p. 76.

By 1962 people were increasingly apprehensive over growing reports about environment hazards. *Silent Spring* gave focus and meaning to a swelling debate and discussion of the issues. The issues involved even more than the immediate and long-range effects of pesticides and methylmercury. They included and still include not only the whole problem of the pollution of the air, water, and food, but also the ultimate destruction of the very planet. They involve reevaluation of the quality of life itself. Nelson Rockefeller said:

> By 1970 we have explored almost every square mile of this planet. We have begun to explore the lunar satellite and the more remote areas of the sea bed. We are planning a "grand tour" of the other planets, much in the mode of a photographic safari. We have explored the microcosm to the smallest subparticle of matter, split the atom, probed the secrets of chromosomes and genes and, through them, the key to life itself. "But with all our relentless searching for knowledge," as Ewald B. Nyquist, New York State Commissioner of Education, has put it, "we have forgotten that man himself is the ultimate reason for our eternal quest, and that the individual is still the basic unit of value in the human condition."[5]

By the late sixties the enormous expansion of science and technology had changed the whole structure of society. The economy had shifted from the production of goods to the provision of services such as health, recreation, and education. The nuclear age had been replaced by the space age, and it was generally accepted that science and technology could solve all the problems. Science, which had been helped by large sums of money from the federal government and large foundations, enjoyed high prestige. Nothing was impossible.

Several new kinds of relationships evolved as a result of the development of a technology-industry-research triad. As the country assumed a more military stance during the fifties and became involved first in the Korean War and subsequently in the struggle in Vietnam and Southeast Asia, a whole new industrial-military complex came into being. There was a marked increase in government contracts with industry for production of military supplies and equipment, and with both industry and educational institutions for research relative to the war effort. A new partnership between technology and medicine grew by leaps and bounds. Developments in medical technology of such things as heart pacemakers, hydrodialysis

---

[5] Rockefeller, N. A. *Our Environment Can be Saved.* Garden City, New York, Doubleday and Company, Inc., 1970, p. 140.

equipment, artificial organs, and hyperbaric chambers revolutionized medical and surgical care. Of no less importance to medical science were the results of genetic research and the development of a myriad of new drugs.

Other technologic advances which evolved, such as the computer, were beginning to create in people the feeling that society was becoming depersonalized. Fear was being expressed about the future influence of technology and scientific advance on the very fabric of life. Some of this was caused by the impossibility of keeping up with the expansion of knowledge. In 1964 Bell[6] estimated that 50,000 technical journals with 1,200,000 articles were published annually, and that major libraries would double their holdings every 16 years. In all of this knowledge revolution a higher premium was being placed on education: if one does not understand what is going on he cannot participate; this in turn adds to the depersonalization.

Population

The impact of World War II on migration was pronounced, and mobility in general was characteristic and widespread. Job opportunities in defense establishments mushroomed, and unemployment practically disappeared. There was a mass movement of Negro families from the South to the North seeking employment. Thousands of individuals and families were uprooted—moving from the country to the city for defense jobs, participation in the whole war effort, or both in combination. Many of these never returned to their original location, and the urban situation never returned to its prewar state.

Immigration after 1930 no longer made any significant contribution to the population increase. However, after the war Puerto Ricans in growing numbers came to the States and more specifically to New York City. The Puerto Rican was handicapped in the American city—more so than the earlier immigrants. His previous life was rural, he could not speak English, was unskilled, and had few financial resources. As a group, Puerto Ricans did not have the cohesiveness and optimistic outlook that was a characteristic of the earlier immigrants.

[6] Bell, D. The Post-industrial society. In Ginsberg, E., ed., *Technology and Social Change* New York, The Columbia University Press, 1964, Ch. 2, p. 45.

In addition to the migration to the cities, there was an increase in the flow of middle-class citizens to the suburbs, and from the suburbs to the semisuburbs. Some of the reasons for this were a steadily rising income level, a better standard of living, more automobiles, and improved roads. The availability of single housing units, better schools, and more common middle-class manners and morals gave a feeling that the suburbs were a better place in which to raise a family.

The movement to the suburbs further increased the plight of the cities. American cities have always been plagued with the problems of the underprivileged, and the situation continues to worsen. Increased migration with scarcity of adequate low- and middle-income housing, inadequate transportation, poor parking facilities, traffic congestion, overcrowding, noise, and smog make the city a less desirable place in which to live. Between 1950 and 1960 more than three-quarters of the metropolitan growth took place outside the central city—and the poor rushed in to fill the void. Poverty, not exclusively a result of urbanization, remained primarily a problem of the central cities and certain rural districts of the country. The conditions of the poor, although not as desperate as those of the earlier immigrants in the slums, were in sharp contrast to those of an increasing number of Americans who by the end of the sixties enjoyed the most affluent society the world has ever known.

By 1970 the population of the United States had reached well over 200 million, and the need for population control was uppermost in the minds of many. Controversy over how to accomplish population control was world-wide.

Education

During the Depression public school attendance burgeoned. Lunch Programs were introduced into some of the public schools in an effort to alleviate hunger and to prevent some of the ravages of malnutrition. In 1935 the National Youth Administration (NYA) was established to provide training for unemployed youth and part-time employment for needy students. As unemployment increased and fewer jobs were available for young people, more and more of them attended high school.

By 1947 practically all the children between 6 and 13 years of age were in elementary school; 81.2 percent of the 14-to-17-year age group were in high school; and half of the 25-to-29-year age group had 12 or more years of schooling.[7]

In 1954 the Supreme Court ruled against separate but equal education for the Negro and directed the states to desegregate their schools with all deliberate speed. There was much resistance to this decision, and the legislators in several of the southern states enacted laws in an attempt to circumvent it. The exact meaning of the phrase "with all deliberate speed" was unclear and was interpreted differently by each individual and group. Token integration occurred, but the majority of Negro children were educated in segregated schools.

By 1970 elementary and secondary education had become a necessity for everyone, and a high school education was a prerequisite for even the unskilled worker. Boys and girls were educated together, both in the cities and the rural areas. However, in contrast to the earlier period when the quality of public school education in the cities was superior to that of other areas, a reverse situation was occurring. The movement of middle-class people from the cities to the suburbs and the migration of Negroes, Puerto Ricans, and unskilled workers to the cities confronted the schools with an almost impossible task. It was difficult to recruit well-prepared teachers to the ghetto schools, the children in the schools came from families that were socially and culturally deprived, and the curricula were not relevant to the increasing number of people in the lower socioeconomic group.

As the number of high school students grew, there was a proportionate demand for college education. This demand had an impact on the expansion of the junior college movement. Junior colleges, or community colleges as they were sometimes called, made it possible for more students to live at home and to pursue further education. For the most part the curricula consisted of the first two years of a baccalaureate program. In the fifties the junior colleges turned their attention to meeting the needs of the people in their own community. Vocational curricula and adult education were added to the offerings. By 1959 there were 390 public and 273 private junior colleges with a total enrollment of 816,071.[8]

[7] Allen, H. B. *The Federal Government and Education.* New York, McGraw-Hill Book Company, Inc., 1950, p. 8-10.
[8] Brick, M. *Form and Focus for the Junior College Movement.* New York, Bureau of Publications, Teachers College, Columbia University, 1964, p. 24-25.

By 1939 the estimated college enrollment was 1,365,000,[9] and the attitude of the public toward higher education had changed. The National Youth Administration with its student work program made it possible for needy students to defray some of the costs of higher education. This was the first substantial federal program to assist students to attend college. There was a growing awareness that the nation's people were its prime resource, and that national security and welfare were dependent upon a high level of education and skill.

The war, with all its myriad demands, mobilized the nation and further emphasized the need for highly educated people. Because of the needs of science and technology, a new relationship developed between higher education and the federal government. The Serviceman's Readjustment Act, familiarly known as the G.I. Bill, which was passed in 1944 is often referred to as the Morrill Act of the twentieth century. To date no other single program has had so great an impact on American higher education. College enrollment swelled, and in 1947, the peak year of veteran enrollment, one and one-half million, or roughly one-half of all college students were veterans. For the most part the veterans were serious students who were more concerned with obtaining an education than with extracurricular activities. Many were married, and their wives and children lived with them on college campuses throughout the country. There was much concern that total college enrollment would drop after the peak years of the veterans. This did not occur, however, as by then the value of higher education for all who could benefit by it had become a pervading value of American society.

By the early sixties college enrollment had reached 4,880,000, and 35 percent of the people between 18 and 21 years of age were in college.[10] The majority of the students by this time were enrolled in coeducational public institutions, with the largest numbers still from the upper socioeconomic groups. However, scholarships from colleges and universities, from philanthropic foundations, from industry, and from the state and federal governments were becoming more readily available, thus making it possible for more young people from lower socioeconomic groups to attend college. By this time the focus

[9] Babridge, H. D. Jr., and Rosenzweig, R. *The Federal Interest in Higher Education.* New York, McGraw-Hill Book Company, Inc., 1962, p. 24.
[10] DeVane, W. C. *Higher Education in Twentieth Century America.* Cambridge, Massachusetts, Harvard University Press, 1965, p. 2.

of higher education had shifted from one of personal development to one of social responsibility. The relevancy of the curriculum to meet this responsibility was being challenged, and students were beginning to demand more freedom in planning their own course of study.

Graduate and professional education expanded, spurred by the passage of the National Defense Education Act of 1958, which provided federal support to students in graduate school. This was the first tangible step by the federal government to ensure that each individual have the opportunity to receive the most advanced education for which he qualified in order to assure the well-being of the nation. Graduate education was becoming a prerequisite for many top-level positions in management, teaching, and administration.

The federal government was turning more and more to the universities to promote specific goals of the country, such as research, training of personnel, and consultation. Scientists and scholars were being drawn more and more into world affairs. However, there was no overall federal policy or goal for higher education as a whole, as was true in some of the other countries of the world.

By the late sixties student unrest and turmoil were characteristic phenomena of the times, and universities were one of their prime targets. The degree of student discontent seemed to parallel the increasing involvement of the country in the Vietnam war, and criticism focused on military-related university involvement, such as ROTC programs and government-sponsored university research relative to the war effort. In addition, student unrest and involvement with the whole civil rights movement resulted in efforts to increase the number of black university students and faculty as well as to develop black studies programs. A general and growing discontent on the part of university students with the country in general, and the irrelevancy of their university education in particular, resulted in widespread student demonstrations, strikes, and frightening violence. Students demanded and assumed much more involvement with both curriculum planning and a widening range of decisions relative to higher education.

The costs of education on all levels rose dramatically, and in many states it was the largest item in the budget, accounting for one-quarter of the financial expenditure of state monies. However, there was much discussion and debate about the role of the federal government in financing and in improving the quality of education.

Women

Participation of women in the labor force prior to World War II increased significantly, but the war itself changed the entire picture. Unemployment was reduced practically overnight, and large numbers of women went to work. As in the Civil War and World War I, they took many jobs that had previously been open only to men. Many were recruited and trained for complicated technical production line and service responsibilities. Others, who previously had been involved full time with their homes and families, devoted their energies to a myriad of voluntary services needed for the war effort. Women for the first time joined all branches of the armed forces and had the same military rank and pay as the men. By the end of the war there were 16,000,000 women in the labor force.[11] This pattern of women working full time did not change, and the proportion of married women working outside the home increased each year. Mowry[12] states that by 1960 more than one-third of the women of working age were either employed or looking for work. Within some age groups 28 percent of the married women were working.

In spite of the increasing numbers of working women, the struggle by women for equality in American society, characterized by such purpose and vitality earlier in the century, was gradually subsiding. No real gains had been made by midcentury. In fact, women seemed to have lost ground in their battle for equality of opportunity. This occurred in spite of the fact that changes in the pattern of marriage, child rearing, and life span had resulted in more time available to women for full-time employment or career development outside the home. By 1957 the median age at which a girl left school was 18; she married at 20 and had her last child at 26. She was 32 by the time her youngest child went to school, and her life expectancy was 79 years of age.[13] There was general acceptance that women had the same right as men to higher education. They had proved they had the mental capacity and the physical endurance. There was not, however, general acceptance that higher education was equally as important for women as for men, and women had not continued to take equal advantage of this opportunity. Some of the women were also ques-

---

[11] Bryson, L., ed. *Facing the Future's Risks*. New York, Harper and Brothers, 1953, p. 193.
[12] Mowry, G. *The Urban Nation 1920-1960*. New York, Hill and Wang, 1965, p. 207.
[13] Newcomer, M. *A Century of Higher Education for American Women*. New York, Harper and Brothers, 1959, p. 214.

tioning the value of their college education, and the early pioneering for women's education had lost most of its momentum. During the fifties and early sixties there was a slow but steady decline in the proportion of women enrolled in programs of higher education.

Of particular interest were the changes in the pattern of involvement of women in the economy of the country, in higher education, and in the mainstream of American society in general. The fact of greater participation of women in the labor force was unquestionable. However, in many instances upward job opportunity was not available, and there were often salary inequities for men and women in the same jobs.

The majority of professional women were nurses or teachers, and most of this latter group were found in the elementary schools. Few were high school principals. Those who were employed by colleges and universities taught predominantly within professional schools of nursing, education, or social work, or were in women's colleges. The numbers with top university administrative responsibilities continued to be so small as to be almost insignificant. A look at responsible positions in government, politics, and professions such as law, medicine, and engineering revealed the same lack of participation by women.

By 1960 it was evident that women had not tried to consolidate and extend their claim to equality from the vote to more full participation in the affairs of the country. They appeared to have a lack of commitment to full-time meaningful employment. The conflict between the goal of home and family versus career continued, and was enhanced by the still-prevalent mores of society that "women's place is in the home." On the other hand, the 1960 society was beginning to change its attitude toward women's goals and to recognize their great potential contribution to a society which needed the best of all of its citizens. Civil rights legislation passed by Congress included the elimination of discrimination in the employment of women. More and more of the material wealth of the country was controlled by women, and their full participation in the economy was increasingly important.

Social Consciousness

Historians say that the depression years were the most disastrous period in the history of the country. There was widespread despair, cynicism, questioning, hunger, and suffering. On the other hand, the depression and the years following had a profound effect on the already ingrained social consciousness of the American people. They were deeply affected by the plight of so many of their fellow countrymen and readily accepted and supported programs provided for the poor, the unemployed, and the helpless victims of circumstances well beyond their control. More people than ever before participated in a variety of voluntary efforts and helped to raise large sums of money for relief and welfare. Paralleling these voluntary efforts was the ever-growing involvement of the federal government in programs for the general welfare, with the role of the voluntary organization a complementary one. There seemed to be a change in society as a whole, resulting in a willingness on the part of the people to invest in the common good, even at the expense of the individual. This shift in emphasis was reflected also in the general attitude toward education. Where formerly education had been considered of value primarily for growth of the individual, its importance for the social development of the country was now recognized.

The post-World War II years were less turbulent than those following World War I. Perhaps one of the reasons for this was that the people were more realistic about the results of war and not as emotionally entangled with slogans such as "a war to end all wars" or "a war to make the world safe for democracy." They clamored and worked for the good things in life, but the social consciousness that had been reawakened during the depression and had changed the whole fabric of American life could not be ignored. The role of the federal government in the life of the people increased, with each Congress outdoing the other in the amount of social legislation it enacted. The distance between the "haves" and "have-nots" became more visible with the nationwide spread of television, and there was a pervasive feeling that the good things in life should be available to all. There was no general consensus, however, about how this should be accomplished. Some felt that the government should assume more responsibility; while others feared too much federal involvement.

National voluntary organizations grew by leaps and bounds, and the generosity of the American people in contributing to innumerable and sundry appeals for funds became legendary. The community chest idea, which had developed after the First World War, became firmly established in almost every community, and the red feather, which was its symbol, became a familiar sight.

"The New Frontier," the slogan of the Kennedy administration in the early sixties set the stage for progress in social welfare, housing, civil rights, and education. The ringing words of the President, "ask not what your country can do for you, ask what you can do for your country," expressed the mood of the early sixties—one of idealism, hope, and commitment.

The Peace Corps gave hundreds of Americans the opportunity to become personally involved in helping the less fortunate in other parts of the world. Volunteers in Service to America (VISTA) provided the means through which people could serve those within the country itself—the less fortunate, the poor, and the elderly.

During the Kennedy era there was a desire for change and a feeling, particularly on the part of the youth, that change was possible. The country was able to take a giant step forward, the greatest since the Civil War, toward equality for the blacks with its civil rights legislation. In areas where federal power could be evoked, government support was received. Sit-ins, demonstrations, and attacks on de facto segregation and discrimination in schools, public transportation, housing, and employment swept across the country. The courage and inspiration of Martin Luther King, Jr., immortalized by both his Nobel Peace Prize and his assassination, touched the hearts of Americans. Larry L. King wrote of the Kennedy influence in April 1968:

> We needed something. Kennedy gave it to us. Call it a sense of style. Suddenly America might be believed again. It might grow young. Its liver spots might disappear. It might reach the moon and other high destinies; young men and women of many races and classes joined hands in the bloodier thickets of the South and sang their hope. We Shall Overcome. Our youth invaded distant lands not with flame-throwers and guns but as missionaries of the Peace Corps. Appalachia would come to life; Martin Luther King would have his dream; America was on the move again. How incredibly naive it all seems today, and how quickly it passed.[14]

The youth of the country were very much involved in the civil rights movement. Their concern soon spread to other issues, such as war and peace, poverty, and basic values of the individual and society.

"The Great Society" slogan of the Johnson era signified the path which the country chose to continue to follow after the Kennedy

[14] King, L. L. An epitaph for LBJ. *Harper's,* 236:21-22, April 1968.

assassination—and extended and expanded federal legislation and support for the elimination of poverty and inequality. By 1964 some of the barriers against discrimination were beginning to crumble, but racial tensions were exploding as the contrast between affluence and poverty came into sharper and sharper focus. Legislation establishing the Office of Economic Opportunity and the resultant poverty programs supported the development of hundreds of community health and welfare-oriented programs aimed at improving services, particularly for those in densely populated cities across the nation. Involvement of citizens in planning and carrying out these services was an important aspect of the poverty program.

Increasing dissatisfaction with the Vietnam war paralleled deepening involvement in the southeast Asian conflict—and the mood of the country began to change from one of hope to one of pessimism. The inspiration of the Kennedy era no longer existed, and an inspiration gap developed during the Johnson era.

Student unrest was growing, and in the late sixties its focus shifted from the national scene to the campus. Campus involvement in ROTC and military research were major concerns at first. Soon, wave after wave of student violence swept across the campuses—aimed at war, inequality, the Establishment, middle-class values, and alleged irrelevance of education. By the end of the sixties changes within the educational system had been made and students were much more involved in decision-making on important issues. There were many people across the country who disagreed with student goals, methods, and aims. Lee, in discussing the college student says,

> Each generation discovers its own gods, its own high priests, its own answers. Each generation grapples in its own way with the problems of war, injustice, sex, and job security and through its struggles with these, each generation defines its own ethos.[15]

By the end of the sixties a deeply concerned, socially conscious America was in the midst of a social revolution and was struggling to redefine its goals and values. This was not easy within a time of an accelerated rate of change. The major issues were not so different from those with which other generations had grappled, but the solutions, to remain viable, would have to endure within the changing world of the seventies and the future.

[15] Lee, C. B. T. *The Campus Scene: 1900-1970.* New York, David McKay Company, Inc., 1970, p. 175.

Nursing

Nurses did not escape the impact of the Depression, and many were forced to join the growing ranks of the unemployed. Their need for full-time, or even part-time work, was desperate. It did, however, aid in the solution of one of the problems which had plagued nursing for a long time—the fact that the bulk of nursing care to patients in hospitals was given by students, with the result that the quality of care left much to be desired. As employment of graduate nurses in hospitals increased, so did their concern about the need to improve the care their patients were receiving. Poor working conditions and long hours of work added to their dissatisfaction. Wages and working conditions of other workers were receiving top billing by some of the labor unions, and many groups were demanding equitable salaries. The American Nurses' Association, in 1946, launched an economic security program for nurses that was aimed at remedying some of the inequities in the employment of nurses. There was much furor about whether this was a function of a professional organization. It was not until the early sixties that the problems of employed nurses were brought to the attention of the nation. By that time other professional organizations, such as the National Education Association, were also demanding changes in the remuneration and working conditions of their members. What began as a palliative measure to provide employment for nurses during the depression resulted in real concern about and recognition of the need to provide better care to patients and better working conditions for nurses. Staffing patterns changed, and the 8-hour day became a reality for many nurses. By the end of World War II the graduate nurse was recognized as an accepted member of the hospital staff, and it was difficult to imagine a hospital without her.

Growing concern over the quality of nursing care contributed to reevaluation of the educational programs which were preparing these nurses. The revised Curriculum Guide recommended that psychiatric nursing be included in the education of all nurses, and also pointed the way for needed reform in nursing education. Changes and improvements were occurring: high school graduation became a requirement for admission to schools of nursing; many poor diploma schools closed; and the number of programs within institutions of higher education showed an increase. The long-to-be-continued controversy over the kind and amount of clinical practice necessary for student learning began at this time.

When World War II started, nursing had already taken steps to meet the demands of the military and the civilian population. The American Nurses' Association, the National League for Nursing Education, and the National Organization for Public Health Nursing early in 1940 held a joint convention in Philadelphia to discuss steps to be taken. Following this meeting the Nursing Council of National Defense was formed with representatives from the Army and Navy Nurse Corps, the Children's Bureau, the Veterans Administration, the Indian Service, the United States Public Health Service, the national nursing organizations, and the American Red Cross. This council became the National Nursing Council for War Service after war was declared. Some of its concerns were to increase and assure the supply of nursing students; to help in the equitable distribution of graduate nurses for both the armed forces and the home front; and to make greater use of auxiliary nurses. It was also concerned about such things as working hours, wages, and living conditions for nurses.

During the war many nurses joined the Army and Navy Nurse Corps. At the same time women in large numbers were joining other branches. of the armed forces. To assure a continuous supply of nurses federal legislation was passed establishing the Cadet Nurse Corps. Students enrolled in the Cadet Corps had their tuition and fees paid and received a monthly living allowance. In addition, hospital uniforms were supplied as well as an outdoor uniform. Many young women were attracted to the Cadet Nurse Corps, and by the end of the war the total enrollment reached 179,000, with approximately 95 percent of all nursing students members of the Corps.[16] Funds were included in the bill establishing the Cadet Corps for the preparation of teaching and supervisory personnel to meet the expanded enrollment. The administration of the funds was the responsibility of a Division of Nurse Education in the United States Public Health Service. In 1944 this was abolished, and a Division of Nursing was established in the Public Health Service and given jurisdiction and general supervision for all nursing in the Public Health Service—another milestone in the development of nursing in the United States.

[16]Dietz, L., and Lehoxey, A. R. *History and Modern Nursing,* 2nd ed. Philadelphia, F. A. Davis Company, Inc., 1967, p. 158.

After the war the demand for health services and health personnel was insatiable, as patients poured into hospitals, clinics and medical centers. Although no overall national health plan had been developed, prepayment plans for hospital care were growing by leaps and bounds. The impact on nursing of new and rapidly expanding scientific knowledge and developments in medical techniques resulted in the assumption by the nurse of an increasing number of tasks formerly considered to be the responsibility of the physician.

Application of continuing advances in medical science and technology demanded a high degree of nursing as well as medical skill and knowledge. Patterns of delivery of patient care were changing, and utilization of health resources increased markedly. People were better informed regarding health and accepted it as a right.

Many nurses who had been in the armed forces took advantage of the educational opportunity provided by the G.I. Bill and enrolled full time in colleges and universities. The number of nurses with a college education was greater than it had ever been. The kinds and numbers of nurses needed to meet the changing needs of society, and how these nurses were to be educated were of constant concern to nursing. The National Nursing Council, as one of its last activities before disbanding in 1948, was responsible for the launching of the now-famous study known as the Brown Report.[17]

Brown reported that persons conversant with the trends in professional education in the United States were practically unanimous in the opinion that the preparation of professional nurses belonged in institutions of higher learning. She advocated that the nonprofessional nurse be accepted and prepared within public vocational schools, that poor diploma schools close, and that the good ones make every effort to further improve their curricula. They should also experiment in simultaneously shortening the period of education while improving the course of study. Especially recommended as transitional steps toward the future were the creation of central schools of nursing and the utilization of the teaching resources of junior colleges. The Brown Report recommended:

> that nursing make one of its first matters of important business the long overdue official examination of every school; that the list of accredited schools be published and distributed as far as possible to every town and city of the United States.[18]

---

[17]Brown, E. L. *Nursing for the Future.* New York, Russell Sage Foundation, 1948, p. 198.
[18]*Ibid.,* p. 116.

This report gave added impetus and a sense of direction to midcentury nursing educational reform. The pervading feeling in society of the need for educated people to meet society's needs was penetrating nursing, and nursing education was moving into institutions of higher learning. Since the beginning of the war, the American Association of Junior Colleges and the National Council for War Services had been thinking together about collaborating further in the education of nurses, as many prenursing courses were available in junior colleges.

In 1951 Mildred Montag's[19] dissertation was used as a model for the development of community college education for nurses. The relationship between community colleges and nursing, at first experimental, became well established as a viable pattern of nursing education. Many of the fears and concerns expressed when the experiment started began to be alleviated.

The structure of the six nursing organizations was cumbersome, and problems of coordination were increasing. After considerable study of the structure of the existing organizations, a plan of merger and reorganization was accepted in 1952. The merger resulted in two companion organizations. One was the American Nurses' Association whose main purposes were the continuing improvement of professional practice and the economic and general welfare of nurses. Membership was open only to registered nurses. The other organization was the National League for Nursing whose purposes were for nurses and friends of nursing to work together, to provide the best possible nursing services to people, and to assure good nursing education. Membership was open to nurses and lay persons alike. A Coordinating Council was established to coordinate programs of common concern to the American Nurses' Association and the National League for Nursing, and to keep in touch with each other's work. At the same time a National Student Nurse Association was organized under the guidance of both the American Nurses' Association and the National League for Nursing.

The quality of nursing education programs and how to evaluate them had long been of concern to the National League for Nursing Education. In 1937 a committee on accreditation had been established in which the National League for Nursing Education, The Association of Collegiate Schools of Nursing, and the National Or-

[19]Montag, M. L. *The Education Of Nursing Technicians.* New York, G. P. Putnam's Sons, 1951, p. 146.

ganization for Public Health Nursing worked closely together to evaluate programs in nursing education. In spite of close collaboration there was much overlapping of activity within these three groups. Finally, in 1948, the National Nursing Accreditation Service was organized. It was responsible for the accreditation of all nursing programs. Four boards of review were established—one for basic noncollegiate professional nursing education, one for basic collegiate nursing education, one for public health nursing, and one for postgraduate professional nursing education. In 1953 the responsibility for the accreditation of nursing programs was transferred to the newly formed National League for Nursing. Criteria for accreditation, and the whole process and procedure, had been constantly evaluated and revised over the years in line with changes and developments in nursing and nursing education. For example, in 1958, the following decisions were made:

1. That the National League for Nursing no longer accredit educational programs which provide specialization at the baccalaureate level.

2. That the National League for Nursing accredit only those baccalaureate programs which include psychiatric nursing.

3. That after five years the National League for Nursing accredit only those baccalaureate programs which include public health nursing.

4. That the National League for Nursing seek assistance of the National Commission on Accrediting to halt development of unsound programs.[20]

Nursing took leadership in its program of accreditation which has been a model for other accreditation groups. It established collaborative relationships with six of the regional associations in higher education—North Central, Middle Atlantic States, Southern, New England, Northwest, and Western. For many years the National Commission on Accrediting has recognized the National League for Nursing as responsible for voluntary accreditation of baccalaureate and higher degree programs in nursing.

Licensure for the practice of nursing was another concern of the American Nurses' Association. The state of New York was a pioneer in this endeavor and in 1938 had enacted a law requiring licensing of all who nurse for hire. The law established two groups—one for

[20]Newton, M. E. National League for Nursing accreditation: From four viewpoints. *Nurs. Outlook*, 14:52, March 1966.

registered professional nurses and the other for licensed practical nurses. This law, suspended during the war, was reenacted in 1949 at which time its mandatory provisions came into full effect. The question of a national licensing system, discussed many times, has run into states' rights as a stumbling block. All states have licensing laws, most of which are mandatory, but there are still a few which are permissive. Each state developed its own state board examination questions until 1944. At that time the National League for Nursing Education developed examinations which could be used by all the states. These examinations, known as the State Board Test Pool, are controlled by the Council of State Boards, which is under the jurisdiction of the American Nurses' Association.

The situation in nursing education was unclear in the fifties, and the great majority of nurses continued to be prepared in diploma programs. Although the number of baccalaureate programs was increasing steadily, many of these programs were not truly baccalaureate, and the number of graduates remained small. Associate Arts programs, on the other hand, increased more rapidly, and the growth of practical nurse programs was phenomenal—increasing from 71 programs in 1948 to 479 in 1957. There was considerable disagreement and misunderstanding about the direction nursing should take toward true professionalism. Part of the problem was due to the small numbers of nurses prepared at the master's level, and the fact that the majority of faculty and nursing leaders were themselves diploma graduates.

Nursing and nursing education was going through a revolution. There was widespread interest in nursing and nursing education among health professionals, general educators, and the general public, as well as nursing leaders. Nursing was planning and collaborating with others on a broad base in an attempt to meet the needs of society. It became part of the Southern Regional Education Board early in the fifties, and somewhat later, the Western Regional Board of Higher Education.

The hard work of seeking answers to soul-searching questions about changing goals and purposes of nursing and nursing education was well under way. Some of the unsolved problems were: What should the role and responsibilities of the nurse be in relation to other health professionals? How should nurses be educated? Why had the graduates of baccalaureate programs not made more impact on nursing practice? Should nursing prepare more generalists or more specialists, in light of the knowledge and technology explosion? How could nursing attract more young people to enter the profession? Nursing struggled to find answers to these and many other questions.

Spurred by monies appropriated by the National Mental Health Act, psychiatric nursing took real leadership both in integrating psychiatric nursing concepts into baccalaureate nursing programs and in developing graduate programs for the preparation of specialists in psychiatric nursing. Federal support through Traineeships was soon available for the preparation of nursing leaders in all fields and for beginning practitioners in public health nursing.

The need for research in nursing was becoming increasingly evident. In 1952 the first issue of *Nursing Research* was published, and in 1955 the first federal money to be earmarked specifically for nursing research became available. As the recognition of the need for research and the development of a firm theoretic base in nursing became increasingly evident, educational preparation at the doctoral level for nurses became both a necessity and a reality.

Rapid changes and developments in nursing and nursing education during the sixties were inevitable and imperative. Society wanted and expected more and better health care. College education was demanded by more and more people and was generally accepted as a base for the professions. The pool of potential candidates for baccalaureate nursing education had increased markedly as a result of the postwar baby boom. Scientific and technologic advances and research had resulted in a tremendous increase in knowledge relative to medicine and health. All these factors converged to support the belief, long held by many educators and leaders in nursing, that nursing like other professions must prepare its practitioners within institutions of higher education. The American Nurses' Association took leadership in clarifying this stand, and in 1965 issued the historic Position Paper on Education for Nursing. Its main components were:

1. Education for those who work in nursing should take place in institutions of learning within the general education system.

2. The education for all those who are licensed to practice nursing should take place in institutions of higher education.

3. Minimum preparation for beginning professional nursing practice should be baccalaureate degree education in nursing.

4. Minimum preparation for beginning technical nursing practice at the present time should be associate degree education in nursing.

5. Education for assistants in the health service occupations should be intensive preservice programs in vocational education institutions rather than on-the-job training programs.[21]

Shortly thereafter, the National League for Nursing supported the trend toward college-based programs of nursing. They recommended an orderly movement of nursing education toward institutions of higher learning in such a way that the flow of nurses into the community not be interrupted. There were and continue to be many within nursing who neither agree nor support the American Nurses' Association position, and the struggle within nursing between those advocating either diploma or baccalaureate education as the base for nursing continues to be a bitter one—far from resolved by the end of the sixties.

The American Nurses' Association grew in political maturity and began to use its enormous influence to initiate, support, and endorse sound federal legislation. Its concern for human dignity was shown in its early leadership in admitting all nurses regardless of race, creed, or color. When a national health insurance plan under the Social Security Administration was proposed, the American Nurses' Association publicly supported the plan in spite of opposition to it by the American Medical Association and the American Hospital Association.

Care of the patient had always been the primary focus of nursing. There was a growing concern, however, about whether nursing was continuing to maintain this responsibility. Increased use of the fruits of technology, such as computers, was resulting in depersonalization of care. Increasing numbers of paraprofessionals and other ancillary workers were participating in patient care. Nursing felt a renewed need to give highest priority to clinical practice. The desire for greater clinical expertise resulted in the development of graduate programs to prepare clinical specialists in such areas as maternity and child nursing, medical and surgical nursing, psychiatric nursing, rehabilitation nursing, and community health nursing. In addition, a whole variety of short, technical, nondegree courses were established to prepare nurses for expanded roles, such as the pediatric nurse practitioner. The need for specialists in nursing to contribute to comprehensive care has been well accepted. The best way to accomplish this is still unclear.

[21] Fritz, E., and Murphy, M. An analysis of positions on nursing education. *Nurs. Outlook,* 14:20, February 1966.

Except for recent years, research in nursing has lagged somewhat behind that of other professions. Much of the early research concerned itself with studies of the occupation of nursing and its administration and teaching aspects, rather than with scientific investigation into its nursing practice. As the number of nurses prepared at the doctoral level increased in the sixties, the content and quality of nursing research improved markedly. Emphasis was placed on the development of nursing theory and on scholarship in nursing, through writing as well as research.

The pattern of nursing education continued to change in the sixties. Table 1 shows the numbers of state-approved nursing programs which prepared students for beginning practice in nursing for each 1-year period from 1964 through 1969. The greatest increase was in the number of associate degree programs, with a steady decline in the numbers of diploma programs. The major contribution to growth was in the practical or vocational nursing programs. The conflict within nursing about the future direction of nursing education continues.

The general picture in relation to master's and doctoral programs in nursing was one of modest growth, as shown in Table 2.

Nursing was plagued by persistent problems relating to: manpower supply and demand; roles and functions; diverse patterns of nursing education; and career conflicts. Although these problems were within the profession of nursing itself, there was need for a broadly representative group to study and analyze them objectively in relation to

TABLE 1

Programs which prepare for beginning practice in nursing
1964-65 through 1968-69 [1]

Academic Year	Associate Degree	Diploma	Baccalaureate Degree	Total Basic R.N. Programs	Practical or Vocational	Grand Total
1964-65	174	821	198	1,193	984	2,177
1965-66	218	797	210	1,225	1,081	2,306
1966-67	281	767	221	1,269	1,149	2,418
1967-68	330	728	235	1,293	1,191	2,484
1968-69	390	695	254	1,339	1,252	2,591

[1] National League for Nursing. Educational preparation for nursing—1969. *Nurs. Outlook*, 18:52, September 1970.

TABLE 2

Enrollments and Graduations in Nursing Programs
Leading to Master's and Doctoral Degrees,
1965-66 through 1969-1970[1]

Academic Year	Master's Degree				Doctoral Degree			
	Enrollment				Enrollment			
		Full-time				Full-time		
	Total[2]	Number	Percent of Total Enrollment	Gradua-tions	Total	Number	Percent of Total Enrollment	Gradua-tions
1965-66	3,123	2,358	75.5	1,279	211	94	44.5	14
1966-67	3,488	2,767	79.3	1,534	189	89	47.1	19
1967-68	3,531	2,752	77.9	1,615	209	105	50.2	23
1968-69	4,018	3,034	75.5	1,766	258	103	39.9	39
1969-70	4,443	3,346	75.3	—	286	170	59.4	—

[1]National League for Nursing. Educational preparation for nursing—1969. *Nurs. Outlook,* 18:55, September 1970.
[2]The total number includes full- and part-time students.

the overall needs of society. A National Commission for the Study of Nursing Education[22] came into being as a result of the growing concern on the part of nursing, nursing organizations, and society in general about ways to improve the delivery of health care to the American people. The commission started its work in 1967, financed by the American Nurses' Association, the National League for Nursing, the American Nurses' Foundation, the Avalon Foundation, the Kellogg Foundation, and a most generous anonymous benefactor. It was anticipated that its recommendations, to be published in 1970, would give new directions to nursing and nursing education.

Public Health Nursing

In spite of its hardships and difficulties, the Depression did a great deal to stimulate the development of public health and public health nursing. Many people volunteered to help relieve

[22]National Commission for the Study of Nursing and Nursing Education, Summary Report and Recommendations. *Amer. J. Nurs.,* 70:286-293, February 1970.

the suffering of others. A large number of these volunteers worked with public health nurses. For many it was their first acquaintance with public health nursing, and they became strong advocates in publicizing the services of public health nurses and in recruiting others for this work.

Relief projects of all kinds were financed by the federal government, with each state assuming responsibility for their implementation. Several thousand nurses were employed in these projects, and for many it was their first introduction to public health nursing. In order to utilize those nurses effectively it was necessary for the federal government to provide consultation services to the states. In 1934 Pearl McIver became the first public health nurse employed by the United States Public Health Service to provide consultation services to state health departments. At this time only a few state health departments included public health nursing in their budgets. Two years later all the states had budgeted funds for some kind of public health nursing consultative services.

The need to collaborate with others in meeting the health needs of people had long been a principle of public health nursing, but the depression and its aftereffects brought this need into sharp focus. The collaboration of health professionals in working together to solve common problems became fairly commonplace.

The Social Security Act, passed in 1935, was designed to alleviate some of the ravages of the Depression. Title VI of this act was particularly related to public health programs and was the harbinger of a new relationship between the federal government and the states. The overall purpose was to stimulate a nation-wide program of public health for the protection and promotion of the health of the people.

There were two major provisions in Title VI. One called for an annual appropriation of $8,000,000 to assist states, counties, and medical districts in establishing and maintaining adequate health services. Some of this money was also available for the training of public health workers. The other called for an annual appropriation of the not more than $2,000,000 for research and the investigation of disease and problems of sanitation. Monies were made available on a matching basis to the states. The amount available to each state was based on population, financial need, and the existence of special health problems.

As a result of Title VI, existing public health nursing programs were expanded, and new ones were developed. The public health nurse became a familiar figure in many of the rural areas where she had been unknown before. These nurses for the most part were employed under the aegis of the existing country governmental unit. Bedside nursing care of the sick, which had previously been thought of as the responsibility of the voluntary visiting nurse association, became part of their services to families, in addition to the more traditional services of health guidance and promotion. At the same time, the maternal, child health, and crippled children's provisions of the Social Security Act were introducing public health nurses to families who previously had not known about their existence.

By 1940 the appropriation of funds under Title VI had tripled. The organization of state health departments had been strengthened; more than 4,000 health workers had received training in accreditated schools; 970 additional counties had some full-time public health services; and 1,150 additional clinics had been established for the treatment of venereal disease.[23] For the first time the United States Public Health Service became a partner and advisor to the state health departments, and through them to the local communities.

Approximately 3,000 of the persons who received training funds were public health nurses. Public health nursing had been included as part of federal and state Civil Service Commissions, and 1 year of academic preparation had become accepted as preparation for public health nursing practice. Only baccalaureate programs which included the equivalent of this public health nursing preparation were being accredited by 1944. Continuing emphasis was placed on the social and health aspects of health and illness as an element of all good nursing. Qualified public health nurses were added to hospital nursing staffs and nursing school faculties. Increasingly, public health field experience was becoming an accepted requirement for all students in baccalaureate programs accredited for public health nursing.

The war, with its medical care program for military personnel and their dependents plus the massive health education programs directed toward the civilian population, contributed to the development of a health consciousness in the people which included the belief that good health care was a basic human right. In the years immediately following the war, chronic diseases and accidents became the leading causes of death; the infant death rate declined dramatically; life expectancy at birth increased to 67 years and over; new drugs and

[23]Williams, R. *The United States Public Health Service.* Bethesda, Maryland, The Commissioned Officers Association of the United States Public Health Service, Box 5874, 1951, p. 156.

vaccines contributed to the control of communicable diseases; graduate schools of public health were established in several universities; the multidiscipline teaching approach in the training of public health workers was widely acclaimed; the Hospital Survey and Construction Act was passed by Congress in 1946, and hospital utilization was expanding rapidly; the United States had become a member of the World Health Organization; and American health professionals were participating and contributing to the development of international health programs.

Debate over the issue of a compulsory national health insurance plan was continuous and gaining momentum as voluntary insurance plans of various kinds became available to the people. Rosen[24] states that by 1953, 59 percent of the civilian population was covered by some kind of hospital insurance. This was in contrast to 1933 when there was only one Blue Cross Hospital Service Plan with a total enrollment of 2,000. Medical group prepaid practice plans appeared and were challenged in the courts by the American Medical Association. A few hospital-based home care programs were developing. These plans made it possible for patients who had been discharged from the hospital to their own home to have all professional and therapeutic services available to them. The Montefiore Home Care Program was one of the earliest plans and provided a model for further developments. The Montefiore Plan contracted with the New York Visiting Nursing Service for nursing care. A few visiting nurse associations were experimenting with a prepayment plan for nursing service, but these efforts did not succeed, partly because of a lack of an actuarial base. The Blue Cross was beginning to set up some experiments in the early discharge of patients from the hospital in order to determine the cost of including public health nursing as one of the benefits for Blue Cross members. At the same time the Metropolitan Life Insurance and John Hancock Life Insurance companies discontinued their home nursing programs that had been started in the early part of the century. The need for a health care system for all Americans was becoming increasingly obvious and urgent. There was tacit acceptance of the fact that medical care was a right for everyone and not just a privilege for those who could afford it. The questions remained about how it should be delivered, how it should be paid for, and how it should be fashioned.

In the late forties and early fifties public health and public health

---

[24] Rosen, G. *A History of Public Health.* New York, MD Publications, Inc., 1958, p. 461.

nursing seemed to be imbued with a concern for how services should be organized and administered. There was a feeling that if the services were organized similarly in each community throughout the country, the people could get the services they needed. It was generally accepted that each community should have a full-time health department. Vital statistics, control of communicable diseases, environmental sanitation, laboratory services, maternal and child health services, and health education under the aegis of the health department were the touchstones of this effort. It was considered that an area should have at least 50,000 people in order to establish and support an efficient health department.

Public health nursing was also concerned about organization. In 1946 a committee of representatives from all federal and national agencies interested in public health nursing issued a statement which said in part that one public health nurse should combine both bedside nursing care and health guidance to the entire family. Organizational patterns were recommended for the communities according to population size. Three patterns were recommended:

  a. All public health nursing service, including care of the sick at home, administered and supported by the health department. This is the most satisfactory pattern for rural communities.

  b. Preventive services carried by the health department, with one voluntary agency working in close coordination with the health department, carrying responsibility for bedside nursing and some special fields. At present this type of organization is the most usual one in large cities.

  c. A combination service jointly administered and jointly financed by official and voluntary agencies with all field service rendered by a single group of public health nurses. Such a combination of services is most desirable in smaller cities because it provides more and better service for each family.[25]

There was general agreement that there should be one public health nurse for each unit of 2,500 people if bedside nursing service was included. One public health nurse to each unit of 5,000 persons was adequate if bedside nursing was not part of the services offered.

Thus, the model was developed. There was a feeling that if somehow it could be adhered to, the public health nursing needs of people would be met. One of the earlier premises of public health

[25] National Organization for Public Health Nursing. Desirable organization of public health nursing for family service. *Public Health Nurs.*, 38:388, August 1946.

nursing which stressed that each community must define its own health needs and determine how best to organize to meet the needs seemed to have been forgotten during this period of preoccupation with the organizational patterns of public health and public health nursing.

It was during this time that the initiative and the leadership role of public health nurses diminished, and public health nursing entered a period in which it was constantly defending its role and responsibility in the community as well as its contribution to nursing. It seemed to be striving to establish a beachhead in which its position would be clear, as evidenced by the concentration on the development of organizational patterns that should be followed by each community. In the process the many forces in society that were operating to make the patterns obsolete before they could become operational were ignored.

Strides were being made by nursing education with baccalaureate programs developed in several colleges and universities. The programs were geared both for the high school graduate and for the registered nurse who was a graduate of a diploma program in nursing. The underlying aim in the development of the baccalaureate programs was that the graduates be prepared for the beginning practice of nursing in any area, including public health nursing. Much of the content which previously had been considered preparation exclusively for public health nursing was now deemed necessary for all graduates of a baccalaureate program and was integrated throughout the curriculum. The community was discovered as a laboratory for nursing students, and nursing educators were clamoring for all kinds of community experiences for their students. Thus, almost overnight, public health nursing was stripped of its content and of the setting in which it functioned. Separate elaborate accreditation procedures were set up for the public health and public health nursing component in baccalaureate programs. This was no doubt partly due to the onslaught of the rapidly changing educational scene on public health nursing and its need to retain and defend its position.

By the early sixties public health and public health nursing began to emerge from their defensive cocoon and to become more aware of the society of which they were a part. Separate accreditation procedures were abolished, and theory and practice in public health nursing became a requirement for all baccalaureate programs in nursing. In 1964 the American Nurses' Association defined a public health nurse as a graduate from a baccalaureate program in nursing accredited by the National League for Nursing.

The contribution of public health and public health nursing to the solution of the nation's health problems was less clear than it had been at the beginning of the period. In spite of the fact that there was a larger pool of nurses who were prepared in public health nursing, the numbers of public health nurses were not increasing—in fact, proportionately, there was a decrease. There were still many communities without any public health nursing service available; on the other hand, there were many with two, three, or more agencies providing public health nursing with many gaps and duplications. More and more professional, semiprofessional, and indigenous community workers were appearing and further complicating the picture. The existing public health and public health nursing agencies were having difficulty in adjusting to new workers and new programs. Combination services had not expanded as had been anticipated.

At the same time many areas did not have any full-time public health services, and many of the health departments which had been well established were not responsive to the changing needs of the people. The cost of medical care was rising steadily, but the opposition of the American Medical Association to a federally sponsored health insurance plan was becoming more and more adamant. Congress was appropriating more funds each year for specific diseases rather than for general public health programs; voluntary agencies had multiplied, and often disproportionate amounts of money were contributed for diseases or conditions that were not particularly significant to the overall health of the people. New health workers, both professional and nonprofessional, were constantly emerging, and there was much overlapping and duplication of responsibilities; and health facilities of all kinds appeared with no coordination or planning for comprehensive delivery of health services to all the people.

At the same time new health problems were demanding new solutions. The role of health departments and of public health in general in the solution of these problems was unclear. The problems of the nuclear age with its attendant radiologic health hazards were mainly unsolved. Noise abatement, smog, water pollution, overcrowding, chronic illness, a rising infant death rate with only a slight increase in life expectancy, accidents, overpopulation, premature deaths—particularly in the young adult male—were some of the health problems to be tackled in the immediate future. The concept of the "community of solution," in which health problems and their solutions superseded political jurisdiction, was beginning to emerge as a method of approach.

On the brighter side, some exciting community health demonstrations were in progress, and public health nurses were becoming involved increasingly in a colleague relationship with multidiscipline teams in providing new and comprehensive services for groups of patients and families. There was a trend toward developing community health programs based on the need of the community, rather than on the services offered by a particular agency. Federal legislation, such as the laws pertaining to Medicare and the certification of Home Health Agencies, the health component of model cities' programs, poverty programs with their emphasis on neighborhood health centers and citizen participation, and comprehensive health planning, were pinpointing the need for a clearer definition of public health nursing and a delineation of the competencies of public health nurses. In 1966 the American Public Health Association and the National League for Nursing jointly launched a program for the accreditation of community health nursing services. This was the first effort to apply the accreditation process to the delivery of nursing service.

By the end of the sixties public health nurses were employed in a variety of settings, such as hospitals, home care programs, mental health centers, housing developments for the elderly, and ambulatory services. A few graduate programs for the preparation of a specialist with emphasis on the practice of public health nursing had been developed, and public health nurses were working collaboratively with specialists in other areas of nursing to meet the nursing needs of people wherever they were found. Comprehensive health service was becoming the major theme with emphasis on the needs of the individual, the family, and the community, and on how the needs could be met with the available resources. The road ahead was unclear, but the period of introspection and defensiveness of public health nursing was ending and a new era was beginning. In this new era public health nursing would be in full partnership with other specialists in nursing and with allied health professionals in providing comprehensive health care to the people.

Summary

There are no key or universal words to characterize the years in America between the New Deal and the Johnson era; affluence, enlightenment, apathy, depression, soul-searching, involvement, and social revolution might each be descriptively applicable. The New Deal had a catalytic effect—making it possible for the country to pull itself out of the depression, and heralding the centralization of the federal government.

The impact of war on any society is always cataclysmic, and World War II was no exception. The people and the economy mobilized and were able once again to reconvert their resources for the gigantic war effort. The postwar period, in spite of problems of economic readjustment from war to so-called peace, produced economic progress for a while, and there was a feeling of optimism combined with a certain complacency about the present and the future of the country. Some of the pervading ideas were:

America was still a land of opportunity and the future was bright.

The nuclear family was the prototype of the American family.

Mobility was a way of life.

The suburbs were increasingly desirable as a place to live.

Science and technology could solve all problems.

Answers to almost anything could be found through research.

Government and private industry must form a partnership.

Education was necessary so that people could understand what was going on.

Quality health care was a right for all.

The federal government was responsible for the welfare of the people.

Between the sixties and seventies a marked change occurred in the outlook of the country. Many of the insistent concerns of the times seemed to converge into a growing revolution of values. Major concerns were: the civil rights movement which stands at the heart of social consciousness; the new frontier and great society of the Kennedy and Johnson eras, with their impact on rising expectations of the people; the emphasis on large-scale planning with increasing federal legislation and involvement; and the legal definition of poverty for the first time. Fears and questions about the future were raised about continued and increasing involvement in the Vietnam war, about the military stance and power of the federal government, and about the priority of war over peace at a time of expanding domestic problems. Pessimism was increasing, and questions were being raised about the basic values and quality of life itself. The youth of the country were particularly concerned. There was a growing feeling that people must be actively involved in making decisions which affect them; that equality of opportunity must become a reality, not just a slogan; and that educational programs are irrelevant for today's world and must be reorganized. The cities were deteriorating, the population was increasing, and air pollution, crime, and delinquency were growing problems. Science and technology were getting out of hand and resulting in depersonalization. Disenchantment with the status quo was spreading. The need for action on social issues was imperative.

Perhaps it was destiny that gave nursing the ability and strength to survive the Depression, the Second World War, and the stressful and dynamic years that followed. Buffetted and influenced by diverse and wide-ranging social forces, nursing was able to respond, to mature, and in its own right directly influence the quality of life of the American people.

At the beginning of the period nursing still was hampered by the "angel of mercy" and "handmaiden of the physician" images, and by the apprenticeship system of education. By the end of the sixties the independent functions of nursing had been identified, nursing was firmly entrenched in institutions of higher learning, baccalaureate nursing education had been accepted by the professional nursing organization as the minimum requirement for entrance into the profession, and the master's degree in nursing was accepted as preparation for advanced practice. Doctoral programs in nursing had been established, and nursing research was contributing to the development of a theoretic base for professional nursing practice. Colleague relationships had been established with professional and citizen groups concerned with improvement of the overall health care delivery system.

Gigantic changes occurred during this whole period, and there were certain times in which nursing had to make crucial decisions—each of which affected its future directions. These times were the Depression and its aftermath, the Second World War, the postwar period of readjustment, and the social revolution of the sixties. As an outgrowth of the Depression, the decision was made that graduate nurses, rather than students, should provide direct service to patients in the hospital. Thus, the focus shifted from private duty nurses giving care in the home, to staff nurses giving care in the hospital. At the start of World War II opportunities for nurses had increased, more nurses had had direct patient care experience in the hospital, and nursing was in a good position to contribute more fully to the direct care of military personnel and their dependents all over the world. Nurses were given full officer status, making it possible for them to contribute on an equal basis with others of similar rank.

By the end of the war nursing had become much more aware of the society of which it was a part, and was better able to respond directly to the forces and needs of the broader community. Large numbers of nurses took advantage of the G.I. Bill and enrolled in institutions of higher learning. This growing pool of nurses with broader education gave added impetus to the need for moving nursing into the main stream of higher education—long a vision of some nursing leaders. At the same time, the level of education of all the people had increased, great strides were being made in science and technology, and the people were demanding more comprehensive health care. The American Nurses' Association, with a better-educated membership, took leadership as the spokesman for organized nursing. It took stands on national issues, supporting legislation on nursing and health matters and taking a positive stand for national health insurance—a position opposite to that of the American Medical Association. It was one of the first professional organizations to open its membership to all nurses regardless of race, color, or creed at a time when many state nurses' associations had membership restrictions. An economic security program for the improvement of working conditions and salaries of nurses also came under its aegis. It was largely due to the efforts of the American Nurses' Association and its growing political acumen that federal legislation was passed for the support of higher education in nursing and nursing research. A further indication of the nation's recognition of nursing as a profession was the establishment of the Division of Nursing as a permanent part of the United States Public Health Service.

At the same time there was much furor and dissension among nurses, with continual debate about how nurses should be educated. In spite of the position of the American Nurses' Association that all nursing education should be under the umbrella of educational institutions, the rank and file of nurses were not completely sold on the idea.

The changes in nursing and its progress toward professionalism occurred at differing rates for institutional nursing versus public health nursing. Prior to World War II public health nursing was the unofficial leader in nursing education and nursing practice. In the postwar years, however, this leadership was taken over by the nursing educators. Public health nursing seemed to have lost its ability to respond to the forces in society that were reshaping the education and practice of all professionals. Its reaction was one of hanging on to proven practices and retaining the status quo. The partnership of public health nursing with public health was by this time firmly entrenched and mutually beneficial. One of the side effects, however, was the difficulty experienced by many nurses in public health in clarifying whether their primary identity was to nursing or to public health. Public health nursing had taken on an aura of invincibility and had become rather complacent and smug about its leadership role in the education of public health nurses, in its working conditions and personnel policies, and in the scope of its practice. Therefore, it was not prepared for the fact that changes in nursing and nursing education would have a direct effect upon its leadership in these areas, and that the uniqueness of public health nursing was not defined by these peripheral elements.

The clamor by the people for health services that would meet their needs, the requests by educators and nursing practitioners for a clarification of the uniqueness of public health nursing, the changing role of government in the delivery of health care, and the increased educational level of the people seemed generally to be ignored by public health nursing, and elaborate procedures were set up to defend the status quo. Public health was also faced with the same dilemma, and it almost seemed as if public health nursing opted to identify more closely with public health and its problems than with nursing and its problems.

Increased hospital utilization, growth of health insurance plans, application of new technology, drugs, and surgical procedures, and new kinds of health workers all contributed to the changing role of the hospital and drastically affected institutional nursing. Initial steps were taken to extend hospital services into the community with the development of home care programs and expanded ambulatory services. These developments were destined to bring institutional nursing and public health nursing closer together. By the sixties the emphasis was centered on comprehensive health care, and the competency with which people met this goal became more important than the setting in which the care was provided.

By the time of the social revolution of the sixties, nursing, in spite of its problems, had made great strides toward professionalism. It was able to identify more clearly its contribution to the health of the people; public health nursing had become an inherent component of all baccalaureate programs in nursing; and nursing was collaborating with others in the delivery of health care, was developing colleague relationships with other disciplines, and was playing a partnership role with others in higher education. The necessity for higher education to improve nursing practice was generally accepted, and graduate programs emphasizing excellence in practice were developing. Nursing had become a force in itself and was in a position to influence the direction and quality of health care for the nation.

REFERENCES

Abrams, C. The City Is the Frontier. New York, Harper and Row, Publishers, 1965.

Allen, H. B. The Federal Government and Education. New York, McGraw-Hill Company, Inc., 1950.

Axt, R. J. The Federal Government and Financing Higher Education. New York, Columbia University Press, 1952.

Babridge, H. D., Jr., and Rosenzweig, R. M. The Federal Interest in Higher Education. New York, McGraw-Hill Company, Inc., 1962.

Brick, M. Form and Focus for the Junior College Movement. New York, Bureau of Publications, Teachers College, Columbia University, 1964.

Brown, E. L. Nursing for the Future. New York, Russell Sage Foundation, 1948.

Bryson, L., ed. Facing the Future's Risks. New York, Harper and Brothers, 1953.

DeVane, W. C. Higher Education in Twentieth Century America. Cambridge, Massachusetts, Harvard University Press, 1965.

Dietz, L. D., and Lehoxey, A. R. History and Modern Nursing, 2nd ed. Philadelphia, F. S. Davis Company, 1967.

Dulles, F. The United States Since 1865. Ann Arbor, Michigan, The University of Michigan Press, 1959.

Editorial, Nursing research—January 1971. Nurs. Res., 20:3, January, February 1971.

Ellul, J. The Technological Society. New York, Alfred A. Knopf, 1964.

Fritz, E., and Murphy, M. An analysis of positions on nursing education. Nurs. Outlook, 14:20-24, February 1966.

Ginsberg, E., ed. Technology and Social Change. New York, Columbia University Press, 1964.

Graham, F., Jr. Since Silent Spring. Greenwich, Connecticut, Fawcett Publications, 1970.

Green, C. M. The Rise of Urban America. New York, Harper and Row, 1965.

Griffin, J. G., and Griffin, J. K. Jensen's History and Trends of Professional Nursing, 6th ed. St. Louis, The C. V. Mosby Company, 1969.

Haupt, A. The government's subcommittee on nursing. Public Health Nurs., 34:147-154, March 1942.

_____Bottlenecks in our war nursing program. Amer. J. Public Health, 33:666-670, June 1943.

Joint Committee of the National Organization for Public Health Nursing and the United States Public Health Service. The Public Health Nursing Curriculum Guide. Distributed by the National League for Nursing, 2 Park Avenue, New York, 1942.

King, L. L. An epitaph for LBJ, Harper's, 336:14-22, April 1968.

Lee, C. B. T. The Campus Scene: 1900-1970. New York, David McKay Company, Inc., 1970.

McIver, P. Developments under the United States Public Health Service. Public Health Nurs., 38:585-590, September 1936.

_____WPA projects for registered nurses. Amer. J. Nurs., 37:35-37, January 1937.

Montag, M. L. The Education of Nursing Technicians. New York, G. P. Putnam's Sons, 1951.

Montague, P., & Montague, C. Mercury: How much are we eating? Saturday Review, pp. 50-55, February 6, 1971.

Mowry, F. The Urban Nation 1920-1960. New York, Hill and Wang, 1965.

National League for Nursing. Educational programs for nursing—1969. Nurs. Outlook, 18:52-57, September 1970.

National Commission for the Study of Nursing and Nursing Education, Summary Report and Recommendations. Amer. J. Nurs., 70:279-294, February 1970.

National Organization for Public Health Nursing. Desirable organization for public health nursing for family service. Public Health Nurs., 38:387-389, August 1946.

_____Minimum qualifications of those appointed to positions in public health nursing. Public Health Nurs., 28:172-175, March 1936.

Newcomer, M. A Century of Higher Education for American Women. New York, Harper and Brothers, 1959.

Newton, M. E. National League for Nursing accreditation: From four viewpoints. Nurs. Outlook, 14:48-54, March 1966.

Proceedings of the Sixteenth Annual Transportation Conference; Salzberg Memorial Lecture, November 9, 1964. Coordination of services—Basis for an improved national transportation system. Syracuse, New York, The Business Research Center, Syracuse University.

Rae, J. B. The American Automobile. Chicago, University of Chicago Press, 1965.

Reinsberg, M. Growth and Change in Metropolitan Areas and Their Relation to Metropolitan Transportation. Evanston, Illinois, The Transportation Center at Northwestern University, 1961.

Roberts, M. American Nursing, New York, The Macmillan Company, 1954.

Rockefeller, N. A. Our Environment Can be Saved. Garden City, New York, Doubleday and Company, Inc., 1970.

Rosen, G. A History of Public Health, New York, MD Publications, Inc., 1958.

Williams, R. The United States Public Health Service. Bethesda, Maryland, The Commissioned Officers Association of the United States Public Health Service, Box 5874, 1951.

PART II

COMMUNITY HEALTH
NURSING PROCESS

CHAPTER *4*

The Scene at the
Beginning of the 1970s

The United States at the beginning of the 1970s is a pulsating, dynamic country teeming with people constantly on the move. The population has reached approximately 200 million and is expected to reach 250 million by 1980.[1] Life expectancy has not changed much in the past 20 years and is 67.8 years for males and 75.1 years for females.[2] The growth in population, caused in part by a decrease in infant mortality, is becoming of world-wide concern. There seems to be general agreement among the people in the United States that population should be limited. The constitutionality of some of the state laws which limit or prohibit birth control is being challenged in the Supreme Court. Federal money, however, is available to enable state and local communities to establish family planning programs.

[1] U.S. Bureau of the Census. *Statistical Abstract of the United States: 1969,* 90th ed. Washington, D.C., 1969, p. 7.
[2] *Ibid.,* p. 55.

There is much debate about family planning methods, and the pros and cons of the various approaches are thoroughly aired in the public press.

The plight of the cities continues to worsen with the constant immigration of blacks and Puerto Ricans into the center city, and the emigration of the more affluent to the suburbs. The ghetto areas of the cities bear some resemblance to the slum areas of the earlier periods. Poverty, poor housing, lack of recreational facilities, illiteracy resulting from language barriers, poor transportation facilities, and poor health make excellent breeding grounds for crime and delinquency. Drugs and drug pushers are flourishing. High infant death rates in some census tracts are indicative of the lack of availability or utilization of health care by the people. In contrast to the earlier periods, the aspirations of the people have been heightened by federal legislation, such as the War on Poverty and the legal definition of poverty. Television also has increased the thirst of the people for their share of available goods. The people are more oriented to the present than were their parents and grandparents (who were willing to tolerate conditions because of the promise of a better life in the future) and are demanding immediate solutions to their problems. Skin color makes upward mobility difficult and increases the smoldering resentment of the ghetto dwellers. The ingredients for a conflagration are present and waiting to be touched off unless drastic intervention on a large scale is undertaken.

Traffic congestion, poor public transportation, rising tax rates, high rents, and bureaucratic forms of city government have contributed to the movement of industry and people to the suburbs. Increasingly, the cities are becoming overwhelmed with the poor, the sick, the elderly, and transients. Consequently, costs for welfare and other forms of relief are rising steadily with no end in sight.

The movement of people to the suburbs, which began in earnest with the development of the Model-T Ford, has accelerated over the past 10 years. As a group, suburbanites constitute the largest number of people in the nation. The implications of this group as a political and legislative block are not fully understood at this time.

Science and technology are in ascendancy and on the threshold of even greater advances. The very secrets of life are being explored, with the discovery of DNA and RNA opening up undreamed of vistas. Advances such as the computer and other technology are contributing to a feeling of depersonalization of society. The compatibility of technology with the quality of life is unclear at this time, and many fear that technology may get first priority.

Larger and faster airplanes are making it possible for people to travel to all areas of the world in a matter of hours. At the same time traffic congestion and poor public transportation are bottlenecks to the economic growth of cities. Passenger railroad service, which has been on the decline for many years, is beginning to show signs of revival. Federal legislation, such as Railpak, has pinpointed the need for a viable railroad passenger system.

Industry, particularly the military-industrial complex which has been enhanced by our involvement in the Vietnam war, has a powerful influence on the economic stability of the country. The conversion of industry from meeting the needs of the military to meeting the needs of the people is contributing to a rising unemployment rate. A substantial number of unemployed are those with research knowledge and talents who have developed the complex technology that is responsible for their unemployment. Powerful labor unions with their ever-increasing demands are playing havoc with the economy and are contributing to inflation and unemployment.

The federal government has passed legislation pertaining to all aspects of life. Funds for poverty programs and model cities, in which maximum feasible participation by the consumer is a requirement, have raised the aspirations of the people as well as their level of sophistication and ability to plan their own programs. The lack of stability in federal funding, the government's apparent misinterpretation of the mood of the country, and a lack of program priorities are contributing to a growing disenchantment with the government and its ability to respond to the needs of the people. Questions are being raised about how a democracy should function and who represents what group. Many are hopeful that making it possible for people to vote at age 18 will bring a new look to politics and government.

The educational level of the people is the highest the world has ever known. Seventy-five percent have a high school education, and 50 per cent of the high school graduates are in college. Fourteen years of education for everyone is being accepted as the norm, and the tremendous expansion of public junior colleges is making this a reality for many. High school and college students are demonstrating and demanding a stronger voice in the course of study they pursue and a curriculum more relevant to the 1970s.

The financial plight of private colleges and universities is acute, and rising tuition rates threaten to restrict private education to the affluent. A large majority of college students are in coeducational institutions. Many men and women's colleges and the private preparatory schools have become coeducational in their own right or through affiliation with another institution. The number of women attending college is increasing after the decline in the late fifties and sixties. It is generally accepted that women have equal rights to college education, but they still do not have equal access in relation to such areas as admissions, courses of study, and job opportunities.

The urge of the young men and women to identify with each other on an individual basis has brought about a whole new relationship between male and female. The sanctity of the nuclear family is being challenged, and trial marriages are accepted by society.

Nearly one-half of the women are employed full time, and the fervor of the debate over whether women can have both a career and marriage is disappearing. There is also beginning to be an acceptance of the idea that perhaps all women do not have to marry in order to fulfill their role in society. In spite of the large number of career women, there are very few in administrative, legislative, or policy-making positions. These roles still remain male bastions. Promotions for women are fewer than for men, and they do not receive equal pay for equal work. Women, however, are beginning to organize and demand their rights. Women's liberation groups are becoming very vocal but are still in their infancy. Some of the criticism hurled at these groups are reminiscent of the attacks on the Women Suffragists in the early part of the century.

The people are involved in a social revolution, searching for a redefinition of values basic to their very way of life. There is a pervasive feeling of dissatisfaction with "the way things are." Disenchantment with the Vietnam war, the ever-widening gap between the affluent and the poor, mounting crime and civil disorder, soaring costs of welfare and medical care, deterioration of the very air, water, and land—all have resulted in fear for the future and a growing, swelling feeling that new ways must be found immediately to cope with these mounting problems. The rising aspirations of the people for better housing and living conditions, employment, education, and health care make the situation even more frustrating.

The kind of idealism which led to the development of programs such as the Peace Corps and Volunteers in Service to America (VISTA) is waning. There is now a new kind of social consciousness characterized by the need for action, citizen participation with the here and now at the grass roots, community control, immediacy, and change. Disillusionment with bureaucracy and the seeming unresponsiveness of avenues for change is mounting. The youth, who have much at stake, are the most disenchanted and have expressed their feelings in a myriad of ways, by marches, peace rallies, moratoriums, demonstrations, and sit-ins. The more militant are using different and more drastic methods such as riots, destruction, and bombings directed even at the very heart of the country—the Capitol.

Definitive tools for the measurement of the health of a country do not exist. When one uses the generally accepted indices such as the infant mortality and maternal mortality rates, the stark fact remains that the United States falls well below many of the industrialized countries of the world. For example, in comparing the infant mortality of 22 industrial countries from 1960 to 1968, the United States was in eleventh place in 1960, and fifteenth place in 1968. At this time Sweden had an infant mortality rate of 12.9 while that of the United States was 21.7.[3]

Medical care, just one aspect of health care, is a paradox in the 1970s. It may be characterized as being among the best in the world and also the poorest. It is in a state of transition. The impact of science, technology, and the use of computers on medical care is just beginning to be felt and may well result in far-reaching changes in medicine itself as well as in its delivery. The frightening rise in the cost of medical care, the inequities in the availability and quality of care, and the appalling fragmentation of services are bringing into sharper focus what is perhaps the basic problem—the fact that there is no overall viable health care system. Left pretty much to its own devices, American medicine has developed into a multifaceted uncoordinated complex within which one can identify two different systems: one for the poor financed largely through public funds; and one for those who can still afford to meet the spiraling costs of private medical care. The financial burden of supporting this kind of a program is becoming unbearable, particularly for the middle-class American, and there is a sense of urgency that something must be

[3]United Nations. *Statistical Yearbook, 1969.* New York, Publishing Service, United Nations, New York, 1970.

done soon to alleviate the situation. Care for both the rich and poor can be characterized as being crisis-oriented, fragmented, and plagued by problems resulting from maldistribution and poor utilization of manpower and resources.

The consumer is very much concerned about his care and is actively involved with other health workers in looking at both the needs of the people and the needs of the community, and demanding more control over how these needs are met. The health team, formerly the doctor, the nurse, and the sanitarian, has now expanded to include consumers and providers of care, as well as a growing number and variety of paraprofessional workers. This expanded team is attempting to design and develop new and better ways to bring health care to the people, particularly to those in the inner cities. Many of the approaches which are being tried are innovative and creative and are resulting in the lowering of some of the institutional barriers to change. Demonstration neighborhood health centers, multiservice centers, model cities health programs, satellite clinics, and store-front clinics are mushrooming. Prepaid group practice plans are increasing.

The government has attempted, through multiple legislation, to encourage regional and comprehensive approaches to health care, with emphasis on planning and citizen involvement. Experience with Medicare and Medicaid has made increasingly evident the almost insurmountable cost of health care and the need for comprehensive planning. Solutions to new health problems, such as those relating to the environment and drug addiction must be found. Many people feel that the government should be more responsive to the country's health problems and place a higher priority on health. The pressure on the government to come up with some kind of an overall national health plan is intensifying, and the debate over what kind of a plan it should be and how it should be financed is well under way. As might be expected, many special interest and power groups have thrown their hats into the ring. The only area of real agreement seems to be that there is need for some kind of a national health plan.

Nurses continue to constitute the largest group of health professionals involved in patient care. In 1968 there were approximately 680,000 registered nurses employed full or part time in nursing.[4] Of

---

[4] American Nurses' Association. *Facts About Nursing.* New York, American Nurses' Association, 1969, p. 9.

this number, 50,492, or 13.5 percent, were employed in public health.[5]

The whole question of the role of the nurse and her place in the health care system remains unclear and is further complicated by rapid changes within the system itself. Direct application of the fruits of research and of technologic and scientific developments have resulted in dramatic changes in patient care. As a result many questions are being raised about the need for additional skill, knowledge, and levels of responsibility for nurses as well as other health professionals. There is heightened concern over depersonalization of care resulting from increasing emphasis on computers and technologic equipment. People are concerned also over the fact that nursing has been so preoccupied with administrative and organizational activities that it has gradually abdicated its responsibility for provision of direct patient care to licensed practical nurses, aides, and other ancillary workers, as well as to machines. Nursing is now giving greater priority to clinical practice and professional competence. More and more research is clinically oriented and directed toward development of a firmer theoretic base for the practice of nursing and for improved quality of care. Emphasis on clinical practice has resulted in the development of increasing numbers of graduate programs designed to prepare the clinical specialist.

The knowledge explosion, and resulting changes in medical care, have evidenced the need for a health worker prepared to assist the physician in a different way. Whether this should be a new kind of paraprofessional worker or a nurse with additional preparation is as yet unclear. Special programs to prepare nurses for expanded roles, such as that of the pediatric and maternal nurse practitioner, and other programs to prepare physicians' assistants and other paraprofessionals are developing willy-nilly, with very little clarification about legality, relationships to each other, or to the overall health system. There is renewed discussion of the career ladder concept. There is a growing feeling that many questions about roles, responsibilities, and relationships must be answered in the 1970s.

Nursing education continues to encompass preparation on a variety of levels—a fact which results in much confusion on the part of the general public, as well as within the profession itself, about what

[5] Roberts, D. E., Saba, V. K., and Allen, H. K. Census of nurses in public health. *Amer. J. Nurs.*, 70:2394, November 1970.

nursing really is. The long-standing and continuous controversy about what kind of educational preparation is best for nursing was heightened by the 1965 Statement on Professional Nursing by the American Nurses' Association. In 1968 it was estimated that 84.8 percent of nurses were prepared in diploma programs, 10.8 percent in baccalaureate programs, and 1.8 percent in associate degree programs.[6] Associate degree programs have shown the greatest increase with a growth rate of 40 percent from 1967 to 1969.[7] A few nursing programs designed for the admission of college graduates are developing. Graduate education has high priority. In 1971-72 there were 56 master's degree programs accredited by the National League for Nursing, and in 1969-70 there were 170 nurses enrolled full time in doctoral programs.[8] Emphasis in higher education in nursing is being given to scholarship, publication, and research.

The cost of nursing education, particularly collegiate nursing education, is staggering. Many colleges and universities, particularly private institutions, are questioning their ability to support such expensive programs without additional federal funds. The federal government has assumed major responsibility for financial support for graduate students, and real fear is expressed about the very future of graduate education in nursing should this main source of support be withdrawn.

The first summary report and recommendations of the National Commission on Nursing and Nursing Education, commonly referred to as the Lysaught Report, appeared in the February 1970 issue of the American Journal of Nursing. The report indicated three basic priorities of needs for change in nursing practice and education. These were:

    a. Increased research into both the practice of nursing and the education of nurses;

    b. Enhanced educational systems and curriculum based on the results of that research; and

    c. Increased financial support for nurses and for nursing to ensure adequate career opportunities that will attract and retain the number of individuals required for quality health care in the coming years.[9]

[6] American Nurses' Association. *Loc. cit.*
[7] National League for Nursing. Educational preparation for nursing—1969. *Nurs. Outlook*, 18:53, September 1970.
[8] *Ibid.*, p. 55.
[9] National Commission for the Study of Nursing and Nursing Education, Summary Report and Recommendation. *Amer. J. Nurs.*, 70:285, February 1970.

With these priorities in mind, 15 recommendations were made for changes in nursing practice and nursing education.

Nursing is just beginning to discuss this report and to realize its implications. The debate over implementation has not yet begun. The report, however, provides a blueprint for nursing and nursing education at a time when its future directions are unclear.

At the same time many questions are being raised about the future of public health nursing services, particularly the visiting nurse associations and local health department nursing programs. The costs of visiting nurse associations are rising rapidly and soon may become prohibitive. The case loads consist primarily of persons who are sick, preventive services being the responsibility of health departments. On the other hand, some health departments are including bedside care of the sick as part of their program, and in some instances preventive services are given second priority.

The joint venture of the National League for Nursing and the American Public Health Association, started in 1966 for accreditation of community health nursing services, is well established. Ninety-one community health nursing services have been accredited,[10] and the precedent has been established for the need for some form of accreditation for nursing services within institutions as well as in the community.

Federal legislation, which includes the development of comprehensive health centers, has helped to pinpoint the need for an overhaul of the community nursing care system. In many instances comprehensive health centers, home care programs, and health maintenance organizations have been established outside the existing community health nursing system. Undoubtedly, there are many reasons why this has occurred, but as the trend toward provision of comprehensive services in health centers becomes a reality, new roles will emerge for public health nurses, and existing agency programs will become part of the network of comprehensive community health services.

One of the basic principles of public health nursing is collaboration with other professional and community groups to meet the needs of patients and families. The development of comprehensive health centers provides the opportunity for public health nurses to fully

---

[10] National League for Nursing. Community nursing services accredited by National League for Nursing—April 1971. *Nurs. Outlook*, 19:272, April 1971.

implement this principle, and to become full-fledged members of a multidiscipline health team. This is an age of specialization with many specialized health personnel, including clinical specialists in nursing, participating in the health care of people.

In Part II we will look at the process by which the community health nurse carries out her responsibility to families and to communities. The process revolves around the nursing needs of families and communities, and the knowledge necessary to meet these needs. The term public health nursing has been replaced by the broader phrase of community health nursing. There are many meanings that can be given to this phrase; however, for the purpose of this book, the following definition has been developed:

Community health nursing is the field of nursing in which the family and community are the patients. Although it is concerned with the total health-illness spectrum, its primary focus is on the prevention of disease, and the promotion and maintenance of the highest level of health and well-being.

The Community health nurse works collaboratively with families and groups in identifying their health problems and nursing needs, in determining the nursing care plan, in mobilizing appropriate community resources, and in evaluating the nursing services given. She may provide the care herself or coordinate the services rendered by other members of the nursing and health team.

The community health nurse participates with professional and lay persons in identifying the factors within the community relevant to health. She collaborates in planning, implementing, and evaluating the community health program, and assumes leadership in interpreting nursing and defining nursing needs.

We believe community health nursing involves a process which includes five steps:

1. Determining and collecting pertinent information.
2. Analyzing the information to determine the health problems and identify the nursing needs.
3. Determining the nursing care plan.
4. Implementing the nursing care plan.
5. Evaluating the nursing care plan.

This process is equally applicable to the individual, the family, or the community. The concepts upon which the practice is based, the kind of information that is collected, the nursing needs which are identified, and the nursing care plan for the individual, the family, and the community are different in each situation, but the process remains essentially the same.

The two major responsibilities of the community health nurse are the family and the community; therefore, the process of community health nursing has been presented separately as it relates to the family and to the community. This approach is used purposefully to allow for clarification and depth of exploration. It does not in any way negate the interrelationship between the family and the community, or the fact that in reality community health nurses often work with the family and community simultaneously. Nursing is a unified whole and not a series of separate steps. However, a breakdown of the process helps to recognize how dependent each step is upon the other, how inseparable the steps are from the nursing action that will result, and how complex each step is in itself. The nature of nursing is derived from the health problems of people, and there is no set of blueprints for action that is universally applicable to each situation. Each family and community must be approached as a separate problem. The nursing actions can come only from a systematic study of the situation—this is the nursing process.

We have made some basic assumptions about the practice of community health nursing which must be kept in mind in all the steps of the nursing process. These assumptions are:

1. The nature of community health nursing practice is derived from the health problems of families and communities.

2. The health of the family is reflected in the health of the community.

3. The family as a whole is different than the individuals who comprise it.

4. The family has the right and responsibility to make its own decisions.

5. The community health nurse works with the family in determining its nursing needs, in developing the plan of action, and in evaluating the outcomes.

6. Each individual has the right to good health care.

7. Health care should be continuous, comprehensive, and available.

8. The community health nurse works as a member of a health team.

9. The community health nursing program is based upon the needs of the community.

10. There should be a direct relationship between the priority of services provided by the community health nurse and the priority of health problems which have been established by the community.

11. The people in the community are indispensable in all phases of the community health nursing program.

REFERENCES

American Nurses' Association. Facts About Nursing. New York, American Nurses' Association, 1969.

National Commission for the Study of Nursing and Nursing Education, Summary Report and Recommendations. Amer. J. Nurs., 70:279-294, February 1970.

National League for Nursing. Community nursing services accredited by National League for Nursing—April 1971. Nurs. Outlook, 19:272-273, April 1971.

_____ Educational Preparation for Nursing—1969. Nurs. Outlook, 18:52-57, September 1970.

Roberts, D. E., Saba, V. K., and Allen, H. K. Census of nurses in public health. Amer. J. Nurs., 70:2394-2399, November 1970.

United Nations. *Statistical Yearbook, 1969.* New York, Publishing Service, United Nations, New York, 1970.

U. S. Bureau of the Census. *Statistical Abstract of the United States: 1969*, 90th ed. Washington, D. C., 1969.

CHAPTER 5
The Family as the Patient

The family as the patient of the community health nurse is based upon the concept developed in the early 1920s which stated that the family is the unit of service for the public health nurse. This concept, though laudable and embraced as a basic principle by public health nurses, never became fully operational. One of the reasons was no doubt due to the prevailing definition of health at that time, which stated that health was the absence of disease. Even though disease was beginning to be understood as having multiple causes, it was not clear how the promotion of health could be conceptualized in relation to providing nursing services to the family as a whole. Another reason may have been that the educational preparation of nurses, including public health nurses, was geared to providing nursing care to the sick individual; thus, the individual was of primary concern. Public health nurses, because their base of operation was in the home, became skillful in recognizing factors in the family that affected the sick individual, and also some of the effects the sick individual had on the family. However, nursing care for the family as a group was difficult to grasp and remained a very elusive concept.

In the highly industrialized and technologic society of today with new knowledge progressing geometrically, the traditional roles of all health workers are changing rapidly. Health is no longer defined as just the absence of disease but also encompasses the physical, social, and emotional well-being of individuals, families or other groups, and society at large. Nursing education programs still put undue emphasis on nursing care of sick individuals, but the responsibility of nursing in the prevention of disease and the promotion of health of individuals and of groups is receiving increasing emphasis.

The family as the patient for the community health nurse puts the major focus on the total family and its health problems and nursing needs. The health problems of one member affects his level of functioning, and this influences the functioning of the family as a whole. If the community health nurse concentrates only on the individual and his needs, she is missing the total picture of the family and may be basing her nursing service on some false assumptions. An analogy can be made to someone buying a house. If he only looks at one room—even though the one room may seem to be the center of activity in the house—and then makes a judgment about the rest of the house, he will be buying or rejecting it on the basis of some false assumptions. In the case of buying a house, the main loss may be only financial. In the case of the family, the main loss may be a lowering of its level of functioning as a unit.

In order for the community health nurse to carry out her responsibilities with the family as the patient, she must have knowledge in areas such as: the life styles of families, growth and development of individuals and of families; interpersonal relationships; groups and how they function; the internal and external forces that are always present in any family situation; cultural and religious patterns; concepts and theories from the behavioral, physical, and biologic sciences basic to nursing practice; the environment and its effect on the behavior of human beings; the influences of the community on the values, mores, motivation, and health behavior of families; medical conditions; and treatment of disease.

Whether the community health nurse is employed in a public health agency, a comprehensive health center, a school, an occupational health setting, a mental health center, an ambulatory service, or a home care program, or works with groups of persons such as drug addicts, expectant parents, or members of communes, her major focus and competence is related to the total family and its relationship to the individual and to the community. The nursing process remains constant even though the settings may change.

The definition of a family used throughout this book is one developed by Winch which states:

> A family is a group of two or more persons, joined by ties of marriage, blood, or adoption, who constitute a single household, who interact with each other in their respective familial roles, and who create and maintain a common culture.[1]

The universal functions of a family as defined by Goode[2] are:

1. Reproduction or replacement of members of society
2. Status placement
3. Biological and emotional maintenance
4. Socialization and care of children
5. Social control

The family as the basic unit in society shapes and is shaped by all the forces surrounding it. In this interchange the values, beliefs, and customs of society influence the role and functions of the family. At the same time the values, beliefs, and customs held by the family are helping to determine the direction of society. For example, the behavior of people that is sanctioned by society will influence the behavior of members of the family. The tacit sanction by society, for instance, of the communal form of group living, has greatly altered the traditional child-rearing functions of the family. The adulation of the young by society has completely altered the function of the family in relation to parents and grandparents. Society with its beliefs, values, and customs invades every aspect of the life of the family, such as the age at which children may go to work, and the age at which they are legally responsible for their own decisions and debts. Society also sanctions what is meant by illness, what an ill person may and may not do, and which treatment he is permitted to receive.

On the other hand, the family is exerting forces equally as strong

---

[1] Winch, R. F. *The Modern Family.* New York, Henry Holt and Company, 1952, p. 14.
[2] Goode, W. J. The Sociology of the Family—Horizons in Family Theory. In Merton, R. K., et al., *Sociology Today: Problems and Prospects.* New York, Harper and Row, 1965, Ch. 7, pp. 188-189.

on society, which in turn may influence or change the behaviors sanctioned by society. For example, if families inculcate their children with the value of the settlement of disputes by peaceful means, the pursuit of war by society becomes more difficult. The beliefs and practices of families with regard to the role of women has made drastic changes in the way society views women today.

It must be kept in mind, however, that the forces operating in society and in the family are constantly intermingling and changing. It often is impossible to determine which exerts the strongest influence because of the symbiotic relationship between the family and society.

The great forces of a modern industrial nation, with its emphasis on individual achievement and freedom of choice, have been effective in shaping and molding family patterns in such a way that what might be called a typical American family—the autonomous nuclear family—has emerged. This nuclear family consists of a mother, a father, and their offspring. Its organization is geared to the needs of a complex, urban, industrialized society. In contrast, the organization of the extended family which consists of parents, grandparents, children, aunts, uncles, and cousins is more geared to a rural, agricultural society which is disappearing rapidly in America.

As a small social unit within the larger society, the functions of the nuclear family have become increasingly specialized. Many of its former functions, such as education of children, occupational opportunities, transportation, provision of goods and services, recreation, care of family members during illness, physical and financial responsibility for aging parents and close relatives and help in times of crisis, are being taken over by nonfamily organizations. These changes are consistent with the changing society of today. Women, relieved of many household tasks by technologic developments, are freer and better prepared to seek employment outside of the home as soon as their children reach school age. Proliferating educational institutions, mass media, and communication systems have assumed increasing responsibility for the development of a common culture and the education of today's children. Children have become more involved in individual pursuits, and spend less and less time under the umbrella of parental guidance and authority. Because of advances in transportation, urbanization, and industrialization, husbands often commute considerable distances to their place of work, and thus are less and less available to assume what was once their traditional role—the head of the household. As a result the basic and vital functions of a family which are necessary for the survival of society, such as sexual satisfaction, procreation, care and socialization of children, and the psychologic and physical security of its members, are now highly specialized functions.

Every relationship within the nuclear family becomes more intensified and continuous without members of an extended family available to cushion some of the impact. There are no relatives available to participate in child rearing and to provide counsel and emotional support to the adult members. The relationships and values within the small specialized social unit, which are so important for emotional security and role socialization, must also be congruent with the relationships and values in the larger society. For example, in America status is earned through individual achievement, with a high premium placed upon individual accomplishment. The nuclear family tends to be organized along these same lines with emphasis on the accomplishments of each individual, rather than on what the family achieves as a group. Thus, a child who receives high grades in school, or who excels in athletics, may have a higher status in the family than the less able members. Within this context it may even be possible for the child to have a higher status than his parents. A continuous rise and fall in status is also possible in this kind of situation.

In addition to the forces in society, there are also forces within the family itself which affect its ability to carry out its functions. For example, patterns of interaction may be changed by the arrival of a new baby, when illness strikes, or when parents get old. As a result the family equilibrium is upset, and new relationships of interaction must be formed. Until the equilibrium is restored it may be difficult or even impossible for the family to carry out its function as a family.

It is of the essence that the community health nurse understand the dynamics of the family and all the forces from within and without that are impinging upon it. She then works with this unit in its wholeness and not merely with its parts. She is the one professional worker who has access to the homes of people in all walks of life and who sees them in all phases of health and illness. She has a long tradition of working with families in their own homes and is accepted by them as a friend and a helping person. At the same time she must be aware of some of the factors which mitigate against her providing services to the family as the patient. These factors must be examined critically, and necessary changes made which will enable the community health nurse to use her competencies to the fullest in helping families more toward a high level of health.

The factors are discussed briefly under the following headings:

1. Results of specialization
2. Effects of agency policies on practice
3. Influence of medical model on nursing
4. Implications of federal legislation
5. Utilization and preparation of community health nurses

Results of Specialization

The health care system today is under attack from all sides, with demands made by the public for more comprehensive services than are readily available. Much of the challenge is being directed at the difficulties clients encounter on entering the health care system, and the fragmentation of services they receive. It is becoming fashionable to point to the medical profession, with its emphasis on specialization, as the culprit in what is commonly referred to as the nonsystem of health care. However, if one looks at the other subsystems which comprise the health care system, it becomes evident that specialism is a pervasive theme. Services and personnel have proliferated without any plan for concerted community action. Many specialized professional health workers are appearing on the scene. Each professes that the family is his base of operation. Nonprofessional, indigenous neighborhood workers, who can relate to the people in their own communities, are multiplying daily. They also see the family as their main concern.

Specialization of services and of health workers has resulted in the priorities for services being focused on the functions of a specific agency or the special interest of a particular worker, rather than on the health needs of the family. Thus, clients and patients have many insurmountable hurdles to leap in order to receive the care they need. At the same time, care becomes more fragmented with overlapping, duplication, and gaps in the available health services. Many social agencies, for instance, are geared to provide service to only one segment of the population, for example, to one ethnic or religious group, or to one specific age group. Others may be geared to providing only one service, such as marriage counseling, or adoption and placement of children. Similarly, health agencies that have a special interest in one disease category or age group concentrate their energies and personnel in that direction.

The nursing care system also reflects the proliferation and specialization of nurses and nursing services in a community. With a few exceptions, nursing has not taken the initiative for both short- and long-range planning for nursing services that will meet the nursing needs of the people in the community. In fact, the opposite is the usual pattern. The late Congressman, John Fogarty, stated a few years ago that there was no community in the United States that could say with pride that all its nursing needs were being met adequately. The same statement could be accurately made today.

With increasing specialization in nursing, more and more nurses have the community as their arena. They are engaged in various kinds of programs set up to meet the needs of such special groups of people as mothers and infants, poverty groups, senior citizens, and special disease categories. With no overall community planning the nursing services to families become further fragmented with several nurses, as well as other health workers, visiting the family for one specific function. Thus, there is much duplication of effort, overlapping, and wide gaps in the types of nursing services available to the people. The concomitant results are waste of precious, scarce nurse power, prohibitive costs, lack of job satisfaction. large turnover of personnel, and an unclear definition of what nursing has to offer.

Effects of Agency Policies on Practice

Policies are necessary to give direction to the community health nursing program. The policies must be consistent with the purposes of the agency and must also make it possible for the nurse to provide nursing service to the family as a whole. Because policies directly influence the type and quality of nursing services rendered to families, they must be evaluated frequently to assure that the best interests of the people and community are their primary focus. Staff nurses and consumers, as well as administrators, should be included in the evaluation and revision of existing policies and the development of new ones.

Policies that make it difficult for the community health nurse to give service to the entire family relate to such things as: the number of visits that can be made to a particular family; the priorities of the agency program; the category or age group of patients that can be admitted to the case load; the kind of nursing service that can be provided; the length of time a patient may be on the active case load; the working hours of the agency; the kinds of records that are kept; the fee system; the types of decisions that must be made only by the supervisor; and the policies relating to who can render what kind of service.

In looking at policies one must also keep in mind that long-standing practices sometimes have the force of a policy and may affect the kind of nursing care the nurse renders. Some of these, such as the length of a visit, accompanying a patient to the clinic, making appointments for patients and families, procedures in the home, and the method of recording visits, have a direct influence on the service the family receives from the community health nurse. Other practices have a more indirect influence by affecting the professional development of the nurse and thus affecting the service she gives. Examples are the practices which dictate who participates in neighborhood or community meetings, who participates in teaching of groups, how in-service education programs are planned and carried out, the amount of time allowable for pursuit of academic courses, attendance at professional meetings, and the role of the supervisor in making decisions about services the individual nurse should render to her families.

A growing number of community health nurses, particularly the recent graduates, are becoming more vocal about the health and nursing needs of families and communities. They are making unprecedented demands that they be given the resources to meet the total nursing needs of the families they serve. The people themselves are also clamoring for more comprehensive and less fragmented services. Community health nursing must join, and sometimes lead, the growing parade of "risk takers," and change its policies so that its practitioners can use their education and experience in creative practices which are relevant to the needs of people in society today.

Influence of the Medical Model on Nursing

Nursing practice has been defined largely by two aspects of medicine. One is the major emphasis on the diagnosis and treatment of disease in the individual; the other is the unequivocal fact that only the physician can make the diagnosis and prescribe the treatment. This is the model upon which the whole system of health care is organized. With this model as a guide, the education of nurses has been geared to preparing them to work with individuals who are sick and under the care of a physician.

With its reliance on the individual, the medical model mitigates against the community health nurse providing total nursing service to the entire family as a group. The illness of the individual and the treatment of his disease receive first priority. All the information about the individual is given to the physician, who in turn makes the decisions about what the individual's treatment shall be and what he shall be told about his illness. The right of the individual or the family to have all the information and then to make its own decisions is not part of this model.

The concept of autonomous functions and responsibilities of the community health nurse in relation to prevention of disease and promotion of health does not coincide with the medical model and can be a source of conflict. This conflict is apparent in the generally accepted policies which state that the nurse may visit only patients who are under the care of a physician. "Keeping the well person well," a key concept of community health nursing, is not possible in this context.

The community health nurse can no longer base her practices on the medical model, but must accept the responsibility and accountability for making nursing judgments in relation to the health needs of families. She may do this in collaboration with other professional and nonprofessional workers, including the physician. Her nursing care plan will reflect her role as provider of nursing care and health teacher, as well as coordinator of the services provided by other members of the nursing and health team.

Implications of Federal Legislation

As discussed in the preceding chapters, the role of the federal government and its effect in all areas of the life of the people has undergone a dramatic shift from the "hands-off" policy in the last century to the strong central government of today. There are indications of the fact that the values inherent in rugged individualism have not lost their glitter; but there is little room for questioning the paramount responsibility of the federal government in promoting the general welfare of all the people. However, the debates about how the government should carry out its responsibility are opinionated, controversial, and charged with emotion.

The American people are in general agreement that health is a right for all people, but as yet there is no health policy for the nation as a whole. Consequently, categorical federal legislation and funding for specific age groups (such as Medicare, Medicaid, or Children and Youth) or for specific diseases (such as heart disease, cancer, and stroke) is contributing to the duplication, overlapping, and gaps in services and the specialism of professional workers.

Federal legislation, health insurance plans, and third-party payments, with all their restrictions and limitations, are tending to restrict the services of the community health nurse to one age group or one disease category. How to meet the health and nursing needs of people who do not happen to fall into the categories for which funds are available is a problem of growing concern. One of the earliest principles of public health nursing was that the services of the public health nurse should be available to everyone in the community. The application of this principle always varied from community to community, but it was an essential part of all organized public health nursing services.

Community health nursing must constantly keep this principle in mind and take steps to assure that the availability of money does not determine the priorities for service. It is obvious that if all the energies of the community health nurse are used in taking care of the sick person who is bedridden, or concentrated on one specific group, then her services will not contribute to the improvement of the health of all the people in the community. In spite of the many pressures that result from categorical federal legislation and from the demands of special interest groups, it is imperative that health priorities be established that will keep *all* people well and not just cure disease.

Preparation and Utilization of Community Health Nurses

At the present time the health manpower needs of society are undergoing critical scrutiny, and from all groups we are hearing about the scarcity of adequate numbers of health professionals. The utilization of the available manpower in a period of scarcity is also getting increased attention.

Nursing is the only profession that requires its practitioners to have theory and practice in community health as part of its generic preparation. In 1968, 43,759 nurses were employed full time in public health—more than double the number of 19,502 employed in 1938.[3] Ninety-five percent of the total were employed in local agencies. Of these, 39 percent were in local official agencies, 37 percent in boards of education, 13 percent in local nonofficial agencies, and 5 percent in local combination agencies.[4] The largest increase in the past 30 years has been in nurses employed by boards of education.[5] The number with a baccalaureate degree and preparation in public health increased from 10 percent in 1938, to 41 percent in 1968. However, over 50 percent had neither a degree nor preparation in community health nursing. About three out of five of these are in staff nurse positions.[6]

As mentioned previously, the employing agency and its policies and purposes exert a great deal of influence on the practices of the community health nurse and her ability to provide service to the family as the patient. For example, boards of education with approximately 14,850 nurses, or 37 percent of the available full-time manpower, concentrate their energies on the school-age segment of the population. In most instances, it is difficult or impossible for the nurse to have contact with any member of the family other than the child. She may know the strengths and weaknesses of the total family of a few of the children, and have some ideas about a few others. With few exceptions, however, the majority of her activities are confined to the child in the school.

The remaining 25,283 nurses on the local level are employed either by an official, a voluntary, or a combination agency, or by a hospital-based home care program. Each subscribes in some degree to the family as the patient and exerts its energies toward that end. In actuality, however, priorities for services may be established on the basis of sources of funding, legislation, or special interest groups. The educational preparation of the staff nurses also makes it more difficult to embrace the family as the patient.

---

[3] Roberts, D. E., Saba, V. K., and Allen, H. K. Census of nurses in public health. *Amer. J. Nurs.*, 70:2396, November 1970.
[4] *Ibid.*, p. 2394.
[5] Doster, D. D. Utilization of available "nurse power" in public health. *Amer. J. Public Health*, 60:27, January 1970.
[6] Roberts, *op. cit.*, p. 2399.

In spite of these obstacles, community health nurses represent the best single source for providing leadership in meeting community health needs. By establishing a milieu in which community health nurses are encouraged to critically assess their practices and to take advantage of every opportunity to exert the leadership for which their education and experience has prepared them, many of these obstacles can be overcome. A reordering of priorities, and the development of administrative structures which permit the utmost utilization of the competencies of each nurse in community health are the first steps that must be taken. In this era of scarcity of manpower and of urgent need to utilize fully the competencies of each worker, all professionals are reassessing their roles and responsibilities. A better-educated, more sophisticated population with rising expectations is demanding changes in the health care system. Maximum feasible participation is becoming the watchword for many consumer groups. Accountability of professional practice is gaining momentum, with people no longer willing to accept mediocre or inappropriate services. The focus of health care is beginning to move toward the needs of the patient and client as the primary goal; and away from the primacy of the needs of the professional and the agency or institution which employs them.

Summary

Community health nursing in the early 1920s was in the vanguard in broadening the nation's concept of health. It has the potential for the same kind of leadership today, with the largest group of professional workers who have educational preparation in the theory and practice of community health and community health nursing. It has access to people from all walks of life in their own homes, and first-hand knowledge of the health needs of people and of the communities in which they live. It has a long tradition of working with families and collaborating with citizen groups and other professionals. Unlike some of the other health workers in this period of turmoil and change, the community health nurse is still held in high regard by the community and its people. In the words of one militant community leader: "community health nurses still have a chance."

If the emphasis of the community health nurse is to be on the family as a whole, with prevention of disease and promotion and maintenance of health as the first priority, there are some changes in practices (which do not require a large outlay of money) that she must institute immediately. She must: give high priority to the independent functions of nursing and pursue them aggressively; become the advocate for the family in all health matters and keep the total family as the main goal; participate with others in planning community health programs; take leadership in interpreting nursing and defining nursing needs; become involved with consumer groups in the community who are concerned with health; seek opportunities to exert leadership in areas where nursing can make a contribution; publicize the factors in the community which contribute to poor health; get acquainted with legislators and support good health legislation; experiment with new ways in delivering health and nursing services to families; and develop friendships with the persons responsible for the press and other mass media.

REFERENCES

Ackerman, N. The Psychodynamics of Family Life. New York, Basic Books, Inc., 1958.

Blisten, D. R. The World of the Family. New York, Random House, 1963.

Cavan, R. R. The American Family. New York, Thomas Y. Crowell Company, 1955.

Coser, R. L. The Family: Its Structure and Function. New York, St. Martin's Press, 1964.

Doster, D. D. Utilization of available "nurse power" in public health. Amer. J. Public Health, 60:25-37, January 1970.

Duvall, E. M. Family Development, 3rd ed. New York, J. B. Lippincott Company, 1969.

Goode, W. J. The Sociology of the Family—Horizons In Family Theory. In Merton, R. K., et al., Sociology Today: Problems and Prospects. New York, Harper and Row, 1965, Ch. 7, pp. 178-196.

Kirkpatrick, C. The Family as Process and Institution. New York, The Ronald Press, 1967.

Pittman, R. The man in the family. Nurs. Outlook, 16:62-64, April 1968.

Roberts, D. E., Saba, V. K., and Allen, H. K. Census of nurses in public health. Amer. J. Nurs., 70:2394-2399, November 1970.

Robischon, P. Community nursing in a changing climate. Nurs. Outlook, 19:410-413, June 1971.

Ruano, B. J. This I believe . . . about nurses innovating change. Nurs. Outlook, 19:416-418, June 1971.

Winch, R. F. The Modern Family. New York, Henry Holt and Company, 1952.

CHAPTER 6
Family Data Collection

Nursing, in contrast to such professions as law and medicine, does not have a general consensus about the kind of information nurses need to have about their patients in order to carry out their professional nursing responsibilities. The base line of information needed by each physician about his patient and by each lawyer about his client has been agreed upon by their respective professions. The skill in analyzing and interpreting the data varies from one lawyer to another and from one physician to another, but the base-line information each profession has agreed upon remains fairly constant.

The writers, as a result of their experience as community health nursing practitioners and educators, believe a similar base line of information is necessary for the community health nurse to provide proper care to her families.[1] Otherwise, each nurse will collect only the information which she thinks is important. How she analyzes and

[1] Appendix A.

interprets the data will vary from one nurse to another depending upon her knowledge, judgment, and experience.

The collection and analysis of the base-line information about a family helps the community health nurse to assess and diagnose the family's health problems and nursing needs in a systematic, organized fashion based upon a solid foundation of knowledge. A plan of action can then be made which takes into consideration the individual strengths and weaknesses of each family and its ability to cope with its problems.

The information the community health nurse should know about a family can be categorized under four headings:

1. Family characteristics.
2. Socioeconomic and cultural factors.
3. Environmental factors.
4. Medical and health history.

It is essential for the community health nurse to have the information under these categories for each of her families. The analysis may point up areas where further information is needed. Each item under the categories will give some clues about a family. However, it must be kept in mind that the importance of the data in determining health problems and nursing needs lies in the relationship of one item or category to another. The community health nurse cannot determine this relationship until she has all the information.

In developing the items, we have kept in mind that with many families the nurse has only one contact, while with others she may have regular contacts over a long period of time. Community health nurses have always made decisions about whether families have a nursing need and about the number of visits necessary to alleviate the need. However, they often remark that they cannot get information on one visit (although, in many instances, after one contact a decision is made that no further visits are necessary). Collection of data in a systematic way will help to highlight the necessary information the nurse needs to know in order to make a sound professional judgment about nursing needs. We have also kept in mind the dynamic nature of the family, and recognize that the community health nurse who has continuing contact with a family will have increased knowledge and understanding of its problems and way of life.

In gathering data about a family the nurse must keep in mind that no two families are alike. On the other hand, according to Duvall,[2] there is a predictability about family development that helps one to know what to expect of any family at a given stage in its development. Each family goes through each stage in its own way, but each follows a universal sequence of family development. This is true irrespective of where a family is found—in an inner city ghetto, in a rural farm, in a suburb, whether in the North, South, East, or West. There are many internal and external forces operating in a family at any one time that produce a dynamic, changing situation to which the community health nurse must be constantly alert.

The base-line information about a family which we believe is essential for each community health nurse to have in order to define its health and nursing needs may be similar to the information that a social worker, a nutritionist, or other professional worker would collect. In fact, there are many complaints from patients and clients that they have to repeat the same information every time they meet a different worker or go to a new agency or institution. Each professional discipline, however, has a different purpose for collecting the data and, thus, asks different questions about it. In other words, the uniqueness of each discipline lies in the pertinent questions it asks about similar data.

In the following pages the items under each category are discussed, and some of the important clues in regard to health status are pointed out. Following the discussion of each item are some pertinent questions the community health nurse might ask in her assessment of the information she has collected.

Family Characteristics

Demographic data such as age, sex, marital status, and position in the family of each member are fairly easy to obtain. This information presents a composite picture of the members of the household and gives some clues about the developmental stage of the family. For example, if the demographic data show that the family consists of the parents and two preschool children, we know that they are at a different developmental stage and will have different needs than the family which includes a husband and wife whose children have married and started families of their own. These data also provide information about who lives in the household, and

---

[2]Duvall, E. *Family Development*, 3rd ed. New York, J. B. Lippincott Company, 1967, p. 8.

the relationship of each person to the head of the household. Duvall[3] has stated that information about who lives in the family home is one of the three things that will predict what is going on in a family. The two others are where a family is in time, i.e., its life cycle within an era of social change and in a given season, day, and hour, and how a family rates in the community as indicated by its social status.

Each person has specific needs in relation to his age and sex. How these needs are met within the family are harbingers to its health problems. The infant, whose needs can only be met by others, requires more constant attention than the teen-ager who can satisfy some of his needs by participation in peer group activities. An aged parent who is a member of the household can be either a positive or negative force in the movement of the family toward a high level of well-being. The size of a family may have some bearing on its health. For example, small families have fewer health problems and tend to seek care from a physician more often than large families.

The demographic data give some background information about the family that is necessary before any analysis can be done. Armed with this information, the community health nurse can then ask pertinent questions about the other data in this category.

The roles and relationships of family members are less easy to obtain and may depend upon skillful observation and astute questioning by the nurse. One of the functions of the family is the preparation of the next generation for its role in society.The values of the community are inherent guidelines that the family uses in role assignment. The roles and relationships must be congruent with those of society if the family is to fulfill its function. Each member has a different role according to his age group and place in the family. The roles are not static, however, and at any one time while a member is functioning in one role he may also be undergoing a role transition from one age group to another. The community health nurse, because of her access to families in all walks of life and in all stages of sickness and health, has an opportunity to observe the members in their assigned roles and to assess the ability of the individual to assume his role. In some families the roles are clearly understood by the members, and there is an orderly role transition from one age group to another. Where roles are not clear there is apt to be role diffusion with overlapping and conflict. The parents serve an important function as the adult role models for their children. In families

[3]*Ibid.*, p. 2.

with only one parent the role of the other parent is either abandoned or performed by some other person. In some families there is a close relative who takes the place of the missing parent. In other instances there is a member of the household who is not a family member but who plays a significant role in the stability of the family, perhaps replacing the missing parent as a role model. It is not uncommon for one of the older children to abandon his role as a teen-ager and assume the role of father or mother.

Roles and relationships that are clearly defined in the day-by-day functioning of the family may be disrupted when a crisis occurs, such as the arrival of a new baby, illness in the family, or the death of a member. How the family manages when faced with a crisis situation gives some concrete evidence about its health problems and coping ability.

Questions the community health nurse might ask about this information include the following: Are the roles of each individual clearly defined, or is there overlapping? Are the roles appropriate for each age? What role models do the parents project? How do the family members get along with each other? Is there a feeling of family unity or does each individual go his own way? How do members communicate with each other? What is the relationship of the parent to the children? Is one member made the scapegoat for all the family problems?

In her assessment of a family the community health nurse must take into consideration who makes what kinds of decisions and how these are made about the family. Herein may lie the key to the total health picture. The decisions a family makes about the individual member or about the family as a whole are intimately associated with its life style. By and large the nurse has her most frequent contact with the mother. If the father is the one who makes all the decisions in the family, ways must be evolved for the nurse to have contact with the father. On the other hand, if decisions are a "family affair," this may increase or decrease her effectiveness.

Very few studies have been done in relation to decisions that are made in a family. In some that have been done in middle-class families, it has been found that in the first years of marriage the husband and wife jointly make the decisions. At about the time the second child is born, joint decision making is on the wane with each parent having fairly clearly defined areas in which they reign more or less supreme. However, major decisions will still be made jointly.

The literature is replete with stories and stereotypes about persons who make the decisions in a family. In many situations the father is cast as the authoritarian decision maker who rules with an iron hand and of whom everyone is in awe. There are other situations in which the mother is depicted as the decision maker. She is equally as authoritarian as the father but her methods are more subtle, so she is highly beloved. In still fewer instances the family as a whole is a council or committee that has responsibility for all family decisions.

In the nuclear family of today, with its emphasis on the individual and his achievements, these stereotypes do not have much relevance, although we still find some vestiges of them. Instead, decisions are often made by the individual on the basis of his own needs rather than on the needs of the family as a whole.

Questions the nurse might ask regarding decision making are: How about decisions in the family? Does the responsibility for decisions rest with an appropriate person or persons? How does the pattern of decision making affect the family as a whole?

As with all other aspects, the daily activities of a family will vary tremendously, but every family has a pattern of sleeping, of eating, and of use of leisure time. Rest and sufficient sleep are requirements for each individual. Successful nursing intervention is related to a knowledge of the sleeping patterns of a family. The information gathered about the sleeping patterns gives the community health nurse clues about the amount of rest each member has and how his sleep pattern is related to that of the total family. If one member sleeps poorly, the effect of this on the total family should be assessed. For example, if an infant needs constant attention at night, this could result in loss of sleep by the father. He would then be more prone to accidents at his place of work the next day. Carried to its final conclusion, the lack of sleep could have an effect on the economy of the community.

Questions about this item might be: Are the sleeping arrangements appropriate for each age group? Does anyone have a nap during the day? Are there regular hours for retiring and getting up in the morning, or is this dependent upon the desires and whims of the individual? Is age a factor in determining the time of going to bed? If family members sleep together, what effect does this have on them and on the rest of the family?

Closely allied to the sleeping pattern is the eating pattern. If each person arises at a different time in the morning, this will affect the time he has his first meal. Similarly, the last food he has in the evening may be related to the time he retires. In some sections of the country it is customary to have a siesta as part of a prolonged lunch period. This may affect both the time of retiring and the time when the next meal is consumed.

The dietary patterns and food habits of families are closely allied to their total life style. Taboos and restrictions about food, which may have no relation to its nutritive value, are passed on from one generation to the next. Ethnic background and religious beliefs exert a great deal of influence on what families eat, and how and when it is eaten. Food has many different meanings for people and is often tied up with family celebrations and special holidays. Children learn very early in life that they can win approval or disapproval from parents by the amount of food they consume. Many times food is the reward an individual receives for behavior that is sanctioned by the family. On the other hand, withholding food is used as a punishment, such as going to bed without any supper. One of the reasons why it is so difficult for some persons who are overweight to restrict their food intake in order to lose weight is because they have a deeply ingrained belief that they are being punished when food is restricted or withheld.

From her observations of the family eating habits, of the kitchen area, and comments made by the mother, the community health nurse can get some ideas about the food habits. An analysis of the food eaten over a 24-hour period will give valuable information about the nutritive value of the food eaten by the family. Observations of the family members help identify those who are obese and those who are underweight.

Questions of concern to the nurse might be: Does each member, and the family as a whole, have sufficient and nutritious food? How many meals does the family have each day? Which is the heartiest? Does the family sit down at the table together at mealtime? Who is overweight? Who is underweight?

With the increasing technology and the shorter work week, more people have increasing amounts of leisure time, and there is every indication that this trend will continue. How the family spends its leisure time may help the nurse know how best to plan for any health teaching that might be indicated. It also might give her some clues about family unity and the use of community resources. The data about the use of leisure may show that some of the members have too much leisure, while others do not have enough. This may be due to differences in age and sex, or because of long working hours.

The roles of each member also affect the amount of leisure time. The way household tasks are assigned may discriminate against some of the individuals. How leisure time is used can give clues about the individual as a person.

Questions regarding leisure time might revolve around the following: Is the use of leisure time appropriate for the sex and age group of the individual? How much time is devoted to watching television? Does any family member have an all-consuming hobby, and what effect does this have on the family? Does the family have any joint activities for leisure time?

Socioeconomic and Cultural Factors

The information about family income and expenses gives some immediate evidence about the adequacy of the income to meet the daily living expenses. The sources of income are a determinant of the likelihood of extra funds being available to meet a financial crisis. The income also indicates the degree of financial responsibility that is assumed by working members other than the head of the household.

The occupation, education, and income of the head of the household help to define the socioeconomic status and give some idea about the placement of the family in the community, its aspirations, and possibilities for social mobility.

The educational level of the parents is a fairly good predictor about the amount of health knowledge they have, and the probability of their actively seeking further information. Persons with a high school education and above tend to read more and to have more health knowledge than those who have less than a high school education.

The income also offers some suggestions about health problems. There is a direct relationship between illness and the level of income, with families in the lower socioeconomic level having more illnesses than those in the upper income brackets. Those with lower incomes also spend a larger percentage of their income on illness.

Knowledge about who has responsibility for planning how the income is spent, and about any outstanding debts of the family, will help the community health nurse in planning with the family ways to alleviate their health problems. How people spend their money is a personal matter that is related to many facets of the total life of the individual. For example, if a family has a future orientation, it will be more apt to put aside some money to meet emergencies that might arise in the future. In contrast, the family that is present-oriented will be more inclined to use its money for gratification of a present need and not be too concerned about the future. Knowledge about the income of a family and how it spends its money is indispensable for the community health nurse if she is to plan with them about alleviating their health problems.

Questions about income are: What does the amount of income tell about this family? Is it adequate? Do they have any financial assets that are available in an emergency? How much does each of the working members contribute, and is his contribution appropriate? What are the working hours of the mother and father? What is the relationship between income and expense? Is impulse buying or "buy now and pay later" a way of life? How appropriate is the person who makes decisions about the money, and how it is spent? What effect do the outstanding debts have on the amount of money available?

Knowledge about ethnic groups and their culture has always been part of the armamentarium of the community health nurse, and it is assuming more importance at the present time. One of the characteristics of society today is the search by the individual for an identity and his constant query, "Who am I?" This is reflected in the increasing emphasis on being part of an ethnic group, and pride in the cultural heritage associated with that group. Individuals, who a few years ago were exerting all their efforts to become assimilated into the mainstream of American life, are now embracing their ethnic origins, and way of life. The extent to which the ethnic background influences the individual and the family as a whole must be known and understood by the community health nurse in order for her to assess the strengths and weaknesses in the family's ability to cope with its health problems.

Questions she might ask would be: What does the ethnic group heritage mean in this family? Are all its activities governed by ethnic identification? Do they identify with the ethnic group for only specific activities, or do they completely reject this group?

Religion, which at one time was a pervasive force in each person's life, is now the object of much soul searching and questioning. Modes of life that formerly adhered to religious convictions are being abandoned, while at the same time the search for individual identity widens. However, it must be kept in mind that the religious background of an individual or of a family still exerts a powerful influence on behavior. Individuals who have abandoned their religious convictions may still have some guilt feelings because of an early indoctrination to their religious heritage. The community health nurse must be constantly alert to the fact that knowledge about the ethnic and religious background of a family gives valuable clues, but cannot be looked at in a vacuum. She must avoid attaching stereotypes and making generalizations on the basis of limited or incomplete information.

The questions she asks about the information she has collected will help to clarify what religion means to a particular family. What influence does the religious affiliation have on the behavior of the family? What does religion mean to this family? How is it related to the ethnic background? Do all members conform in the same way? How do they explain the differences between their behavior and their religious teachings? If the parents have different religious backgrounds, how is this affecting the family?

Probably the most important determinant of how people behave is related to their value system and what they believe is important and unimportant. For example, if one believes in education, he makes sure his sons and daughters have an education; if he believes prevention of disease is important, he will get his children immunized; and if he believes that owning his own home is important, he will strive toward that goal. It is not possible for the community health nurse to have an understanding of the value system of a family on one contact. However, she can get some clues from the comments of the mother, her observations of the furniture in the home, its condition, the housecleaning, the kind of clothing worn by each member, the make of the automobile they own, the state of repairs inside and outside of the home, and the type of neighborhood in which the family lives. The values of a family are closely associated with its life style and aspirations.

The community health nurse has her own hierarchies of values that have a similar influence on her way of thinking and behaving. In order for any nursing intervention to be effective, she must maintain a constant vigil to avoid making judgments about the family based on what she believes is right and wrong. However, having knowledge and understanding about the value system of a family, assessing its strengths and weaknesses in relation to its values, and working with the family within this system does not mean that the community health nurse has to abandon her own values and embrace those of the family with whom she is working. Her professional responsibility is to help families recognize their health problems, and to provide the necessary information and assistance that will enable them to make sound decisions about the alleviation or solution of these problems.

Examples of questions she might ask about the information are: What is the relation of the value system to the ethnic background and religion of the family? How are discrepancies handled? What seem to be the positive values? What about the negative ones?

The family is only one of the many institutions and resources within a community. The autonomous nuclear family, with its limited contact and responsibility for extended family members, is dependent upon extrafamilial agencies, instituions, and social contacts in order to maintain itself. Significant others, such as close friends and neighbors, become important extensions of the family and lend help and assistance in time of need. The relationship of each family to the larger community gives some indication of its place in society as a whole and of the extrafamilial resources that are utilized. Some families have only superficial and limited contact with programs or institutions in the community, and tend to be alienated from anything other than the immediate family and its problems. Others become so completely involved in community activities that home becomes just a place to sleep and to have an occasional meal; while still others seem to have the ability to enrich the quality of life of the family as a unit by the judicious use of community agencies and participation in their activities. Knowledge of the extent of societal contacts helps the community health nurse in her assessment of the strengths and weaknesses of the family's ability to cope with its health problems.

She may ask herself these questions: What does the participation of the family in community agencies tell one about this family? Is it tied in with their ethnic heritage and religious background? Are there significant others, and what effect do they have on the family? Do all members participate in some community activity? Is it appropriate for each member's age and sex?

Environmental Factors

Shelter is one of the basic needs of all people, and the type and kind of housing play an important part in the life of the family. Housing also affects health, as there is a direct relationship between the kind of housing and the health problems of a family. This is particularly evident in the incidence of illness and disability in children, with a much higher incidence found in those living under poor housing circumstances. The observations of the community health nurse about the living space, the sleeping arrangements, the adequacy of the furniture, the type of refrigeration, the toilet facilities, the presence or absence of flies and rodents, the water supply, and the internal and external accident hazards give valuable insight into what some of the health problems may be and how the family copes with them.

In the assessment of the environmental factors, the information about the type and quality of housing should be looked at in relation to the effect on the particular family. Are the living space, furniture, refrigeration, and toilet facilities adequate? Are the accident hazards due to improper care of the house by the landlord, or are they due to misuse of the property by the family? Does the condition of the dwelling conform to the housing regulations in the community? What clues are available as to possible health problems?

The neighborhood and community in which a family lives exert a tremendous influence on the family. In turn, the family is the bridge to the organizations and activities in the community. The influence of the community is seen in the type of dwellings and how they are kept up; the use of health and related facilities; the buying patterns of the people; the feelings about the schools; the incidence of crime; and the way the people view the police and other protective services, to name a few.

Health facilities, social and welfare agencies, recreation areas, and churches may be available in the community, but they may not be utilized by the family because public transportation is inconvenient or inaccessible. Transportation, which has played so important a part in the development of the country since 1865, is still making tremendous strides in transporting people from one section of the world to another. However, an impasse seems to have been reached in public transportation systems in the urban and suburban areas, with less service available each year.

How people feel about using the available community facilities has a great deal to do with their experiences in using neighborhood agencies or institutions. If the experiences have been positive, the use will be greater than if they were dissatisfied with their previous encounters. These feelings may have no relationship to the quality of the program and services offered by the agency or institution.

The total environment of the individual and family is receiving increased emphasis today, and cannot be ignored in assessing the health and nursing needs of families. One cannot identify and treat the health problems of a family without understanding its environment and the effect on the individual and family. The "community of solution" for the majority of health problems of families probably lies in their own neighborhood and the milieu from which the problems developed and were nurtured.

Assessment of the environmental information would include some of the following questions: In what kind of neighborhood does the family live? How do the type and the condition of the housing of the family compare with other dwellings in the neighborhood? Is there pressure from the neighborhood for all families to conform to one standard? If health and social facilities are available, are they used? If public transportation is not available, what other means are used to transport the people?

Health and Medical History   The standards of health in a family come from its own background, history, and tradition. The health practices vary from family to family, but there are some common characteristics. The knowledge a family has about health and the value it puts upon it are important determinants for its health behavior. Health is an abstract term that has many different meanings. It is something that everyone is for, but a clear-cut definition eludes them. By and large, if health is thought of at all, it is related to the absence of disease. It is necessary for the nurse to understand the meaning of health to a family in order to determine what it perceives to be its health problems. Perhaps it will be necessary to broaden the family's definition of health before any nursing intervention can be implemented.

Questions which will help in assessing the information are: What is the relationship of the health practices of the family to its knowledge and attitude about health? How accurate is its definition of its health problems?

The medical history of each family member should be obtained in order to have information about the past and present significant illnesses for which medical care was sought. The current illnesses and any treatment and medications being taken should be ascertained.

The presence of acute or chronic disease in one member of a family can change the balance of the many forces that are operating at any one time and can cause temporary or permanent disruption in the family.

Some idea about what the family thinks about disease prevention can be arrived at by the immunization status of each individual. When and why a member visits the physician adds to the clues about the value placed on prevention of disease.

The nurse in assessing this information might ask: What is the present state of illness in each member? What relation does the treatment and medication he is receiving have to his present illness? Is the immunization status of each person up to date?

Families today are victims of a maze of health care services and facilities. The specialism in medicine makes it virtually impossible to obtain a family physician, and patients are shuttled back and forth from one specialist to another. One of the ironies of this affluent country in the latter third of the twentieth century is that hospital emergency rooms are replacing the family physician. The high cost of medical and dental care is also one of the deterrents to seeking help. The method of paying for medical care is an important factor to be kept in mind in assessing family health needs.

Questions related to medical care might include: What is the source of medical care for the family? Is it different for each individual? What effect does the cost of medical care have on the utilization of physicians' services? Does the health insurance, if any, include the entire family? Are preventive services included?

How the family manages and where and to whom it turns for help in time of illness or crisis must be included in the base-line information. Relatives or adult family members may be the resource that is used. In some situations neighbors and close friends are the source of help. It is being recognized more and more today that there are specific persons outside the immediate family constellation who exert a considerable amount of influence on the behavior of the individual members and on the family as a whole. These persons are referred to as significant others.

Related questions are: What influence does the source of help the family seeks have on the family? Is it appropriate? How important to the family are the "significant others?" How consistent is the pattern of managing in time of illness or crisis? Is this a source of strength in the present situation?

How individuals perceive the role of health professionals will influence the utilization and value they place upon the services. The past experiences the family has had with a community health nurse and the outcomes of the experiences will influence the expectations it has of her services. If, for example, its only experience was the help she rendered when a new baby arrived, or the weekly bath she gave to the grandmother, its knowledge of the scope of her services will be limited to these areas.

Why does the family think the community health nurse is visiting, and what does it think she can or will do? Community health nurses often fail to ask these kinds of questions and thus do not know how they are perceived by the family. In reality, however, these may be the most important questions the nurse can ask if she hopes to work with the family in developing a plan for nursing intervention. How does its expectations of the services it wants from the community health nurse coincide with the accepted functions? What is the difference between its perception of its nursing problems and the perceptions of the community health nurse?

The preceding discussion has dealt with the importance of systematic collection of base-line information about families in order for the community health nurse to define the health problems and identify the nursing needs. The kinds of information needed and the clues to be garnered from it have been pointed out. The analysis of this information for the identification of nursing needs is explored in the next chapter.

REFERENCES

Ackerman, N. The Psychodynamics of Family Life. New York, Basic Books, 1958.

Black, K., Sr. Teaching family process and intervention. Nurs. Outlook, 18:54-58, June 1970.

Duvall, E. Family Development, 3rd ed. New York, J. B. Lippincott Company, 1967.

Hall, M., and Lefson, E. Family Centered Public Health Nursing. League Exchange No. 39. New York, National League for Nursing, 1959.

Kirkpatrick, C. The Family as Process and Institution. New York, The Ronald Press, 1955.

Levine, M. Adaptation and assessment. A rationale for nursing intervention. Amer. J. Nurs., 66:2450-2453, November 1966.

Pollock, O. A family diagnosis model. Social Service Rev., 34:19-31, March 1969.

Poston, R. Comparative Community Organization. In Duhl, L., ed., The Urban Condition. New York, Simon and Schuster, 1969, Ch. 24, pp. 311-318.

Wilmer, D., and Walkley, R. Effects of Housing on Health and Housing. In Duhl, L., ed., The Urban Condition. New York, Simon and Schuster, 1969. Ch. 16. pp. 215-228.

CHAPTER 7

Analysis of Data and Identification of Family Nursing Needs

Nursing has not as yet developed a specific conceptual framework that provides a theoretic base for the study of the health problems and nursing needs of families. Various concepts and theories from the behavioral, physical, and biologic sciences are being tested for their relevance to nursing. Some of the approaches used by other disciplines in studying families that may have significance for nursing have been summarized by Hill and Hansen.[1]

1. The *interaction approach* views the family as a unity of interacting persons. Each person has a position in the family in which he perceives the norms or role expectations held by other individuals (or by the family as a whole) as the basis for his attitudes and behavior. In any situation the individual will define his role expectations primarily in light of their source and his own self-conception. Then he role plays. The family is studied through analyzing the interac-

---

[1]Hill, R., and Hansen, D. The identification of conceptual frameworks utilized in family study. *Marriage and Family Living*, 22:299-311, November 1960.

tions of the role-playing members. The focus is on the internal structure of the family but neglects the family and its relation to the community.

2. The *structure-function approach* views the family as a social system and one of the many components of the complete social system—or society. The family has functions to perform in society. The family is composed of individuals who are significant for their functions in the maintenance of the family system, and ultimately the social system. Individuals contribute to the boundary maintenance of the system by acting either in response to the demands or constraints of the structure. The scope is broad and could include the interplay of the family and other systems in society as well as the transactions between the family members. The emphasis, however, has been on the statics of structure with a concomitant neglect of change and dynamics.

3. The *situational approach* is based on the assumption that all behavior is purposive in relation to the situation that triggered it. The individual reacts to the crisis or problem which the situation presents on the basis of how he perceives it, and his previous experience in other situations. The situation itself, or the individual's behavior in the situation, is the focus for the study of families.

4. The *institutional approach* emphasizes the family as a social unity in which the individual and cultural values are the main concern. The individual's values and learned needs are transmitted from one generation to the next within the individual family systems. These family systems and the cultural milieu in which the family exists comprise the situation.

5. The *developmental approach* has as its focus the study of the developmental phases of the family from the wedding to old age, and finally the dissolution of the family through death. The changing developmental tasks and role expectations of parents and children as they go through the family life cycle, as well as the developmental tasks of the family as a whole, are the basis for this approach. Generalizations about internal developments of families can be made with this approach.

On the basis of recent findings in nursing research, some of the limitations in using conceptual frameworks from other disciplines in the development of nursing theory have become apparent. There is a growing feeling among nursing researchers that nursing theory must come, at least in part, from the actual practice of nursing, and that it must be tested by actual nursing experience. Community health nurses, because of their close relationships with families, have the opportunity to be in the vanguard in conceptualizing the process of providing nursing services to the family as the patient, and at the same time adding to the general theories about families.

In this chapter each of the types of information collected about the family has been categorized according to whether it is most pertinent in defining the family health problems, in developing the family nursing care plan, or implementing the family nursing care plan. The items under each category are shown in Table 1.

TABLE 1

Family information most relevant to defining health problems
and developing and implementing the nursing care plan

Defining Family Health Problems	Developing Family Nursing Care plan	Implementing Family Nursing Care Plan
Accident Hazards	Education	Availability and Accessibility
Current Illnesses	Ethnic Background and	of Health Facilities
Demographic Data	Religious Practices	Expectations of Services of
Eating Patterns	Health Knowledge	Community Health Nurse
Food Storage	Health Practices	Participation in Community
Living Space	Health Problems as Seen	Activities
Medical History	by Family	Past Experiences with Health
of Each Individual	Health Problems as Seen	Professionals
Rodents and Flies	by Nurse	Relationship of Family to
Sleeping Arrangements	Income and Expenses	Larger Community
Sleeping Patterns	Medical and Dental Care	Role Assignment
Toilet Facilities	Pattern of Decision	Role Model of Parents
Treatment and	Making	Sources of Help Used by
Medicines	Relationships of Members	Family
Water Supply	to Each Other	Transportation Facilities
	Type of Neighborhood	Use of Community Agencies
	Use of Leisure	Value System

This approach is not based on any one conceptual framework. It is, rather, a method of organizing the data in such a way that the relationship of the items to each other and to the family information can be clarified and better understood. The authors are aware of the pitfalls inherent in the analysis of the information in this way. However, we believe that by pinpointing the information most pertinent to the definition of health problems and nursing needs, to the development of the nursing care plan, and to the implementation of the plan, and by discussing this information in relation to each category, that the usefulness and value of the data will be enhanced.

It has been mentioned previously that the steps in the nursing process are interdependent and that one or more steps may occur simultaneously. Similarly, the items and categories of the base-line information are not discrete entities in relation to the steps involved in the analysis of data. They are characterized by the interrelatedness of cause and effect, and cannot be looked at in isolation. At any one time the impact of an item or items may be greater in one aspect of the process than in another. The meaning of the interrelatedness of all the information in relation to the health of the total family and the resultant nursing needs is dependent upon the nursing skill, knowledge, and judgment of the community health nurse.

The items most directly related to developing the family nursing care plan are:

Education

Ethnic and religious practices

Health knowledge

Health practices

Health problems as seen by family

Health problems as seen by nurse

Income and expenses

Medical and dental care

Method of payment for medical and dental care

Pattern of decision making

Relation of members to each other

Type of neighborhood

Use of leisure

The nursing care plan is the blueprint for nursing action in the family. It is based upon the nursing needs and contains the short- and long-range goals for the family that can be accomplished by nursing intervention.

The relationships of family members to each other, although they influence the definition of the health problem, have a greater impact on the kind of nursing care plan that is developed. For example, a family in which each member helps the others, and in which there is a feeling of family unity, requires a different kind of nursing care plan than a family in which these aspects are not present.

How decisions are made in a family may be one of the key aspects of the nursing care plan. Too often, the decision-making apparatus of a family is bypassed in this step of the nursing process. The end result is that the health behavior necessary to meet the nursing goals is not sanctioned by the family and does not become operational, in spite of the efforts of the community health nurse.

The items relating to education, income, expenses, and the ethnic background and religious practices, while playing a role in determining health problems, exert a greater influence on the kind of nursing care plan which evolves. For example, the amount and kind of health teaching is determined by the educational level of the family; the ethnic background and religious practices also influence the kind and amount of health teaching that is necessary and acceptable to the family. The income and expenses influence all aspects and may be one of the more important determinants of the final plan and its implementation and outcomes.

The knowledge the family has about health, and the pattern of health practices are integral parts of the nursing plan. The core of the plan may be to correct some of the health misinformation and to change some of the health practices. The type of medical and dental care and the method of payment must not be ignored. The American people subscribe to the fact that good health care is a right of every individual, but the kind and amount of health care received often depends upon the economic status of the individual or family. What the family perceives as its health problems may not be what the nurse sees. These differences, if any, must be resolved as the plan is developed.

The type of neighborhood and its influence on the family also exert an influence on the successful development of the nursing action. The mores of the neighborhood, such as the upkeep of the dwellings, the way people view the police or other protective services, the waste disposal system, and the schools and churches, tend to force a general pattern of conformity on the families. The nursing care plan must be consistent with this pattern.

The items which are most directly related to implementing the family nursing care plan are:

> Availability and accessibility of health facilities
> Expectations of services from the community health nurse
> Participation in community activities
> Past experience with health professionals
> Relationship of family to larger community

Role assignment of family members
Role model of parents
Sources of help used by the family
Transportation and facilities
Use of community agencies
Value system

Unless the nursing care plan can be implemented, the whole process up to this point becomes an intellectual exercise, or as some say, "an exercise in futility." The implementation of the plan is what the nursing process is all about—carrying out the nursing action based upon the identified nursing needs.

The items that take precedence in this step of the process are the ones relating to the resources the family uses in time of illness or crisis, its past experience with health professionals and community health nurses and its expectations of services from the community health nurse. The information relating to these items gives many clues about the ability of the family to cope with its health problems and which situations will require outside assistance. The family's past experiences with health professionals and community health nurses color its expectations about the activities which can be carried out in its present situation.

The roles each member assumes and their appropriateness are important for implementing the nursing care plan. This is also true of the adult role models the parents present. It may be that the nursing action will require additional functions to be added to the current role assignments.

The value system of the family, a strong determinant of its behavior, exerts a strong influence on the implementation of the plan. This is also true of the items relating to the relationships of the family to the larger community, and its participation or nonparticipation in the extrafamily institutions and organizations.

The availability of health and related facilities in the neighborhood, and the use and nonuse of these by the family, help in understanding this phase of the nursing process. The facilities may be utilized because of the prevailing mores of the neighborhood, but their accessibility is also an important factor. If people cannot reach the resources because transportation is inadequate, inconvenient, or nonexistent, the facilities will not be used irrespective of the quality of services offered.

Identifying Family Nursing
Needs

The steps in the nursing process are characterized by their
interrelatedness, with no even
flow from one step to another.
There is, however, a developmental aspect to the whole process, with
each step dependent upon the other. The analysis of the base-line
information to identify the family nursing needs is probably the
most important step in the nursing process, as the identified needs
form the basis for the nursing actions which ensue. Thus, if the needs
are identified incorrectly, the remaining steps are meaningless, and
the resultant nursing action may be ineffective or even detrimental to
the family.

Throughout this book the authors have defined a nursing need as
the contribution nursing can make to the solution of a health
problem. From many sources today the terms *nursing diagnosis* and
nursing prognosis are used quite frequently when nursing and the
nursing process are being discussed. There is no general agreement
about the definition of these terms or of their meaning in relation to
nursing. Each discussant uses them within his own frame of reference. Because of the confusion in the definition of the terms, their
connotation to disease conditions, and the lack of a nomenclature
for nursing situations, the writers have refrained from using them.

The base-line information about the family may be collected by
the nurse or by other members of the health team. The community
health nurse, however, has the responsibility for analyzing the information to determine the contribution of nursing to the solution of
family health problems. Health encompasses the physical, social, and
emotional well-being of a family and exerts a strong influence on its
ability to carry out its functions.

The first consideration of the nurse is the analysis of the data to
determine the family health problems. The nursing needs of the
family are then identified from the health problems. A family or a
community may have a health problem for which there can be many
nursing needs. On the other hand, there can be several health problems for which there are no nursing needs. The contribution of
nursing to the solution of the health problem may take several
different forms depending upon the needs of the family. For example, in some instances the nurse may help the family to cope more
effectively with a present problem, while in another situation she
may help to prevent a problem from occurring. The nursing actions

will include such things as anticipatory guidance, health teaching, health counseling, and referral, as well as direct nursing care. Her primary focus is the prevention of disease and the promotion and maintenance of health for ultimate high-level well-being.

The family information most pertinent to defining family health problems is shown in Table 2.

TABLE 2

**Items directly related to defining
family health problems**

Accident hazards
Current illnesses
Demographic data
Eating patterns
Food storage
Living space
Medical history of each individual
Rodents and flies
Sleeping arrangements
Sleeping patterns
Toilet facilities
Treatments and medications
Water supply

Clues about the presence of possible health problems can be garnered from these data. These clues also give leads for areas in which further investigation is necessary. For example, the demographic data, which includes information about the number of persons in the household, age, sex, and so forth, may indicate social or emotional problems related to overcrowding and lack of privacy. This item may also point out a problem of fertility or infertility in which family planning is a major need. Nutritional practices which contribute to health problems can be ascertained by the information about family eating patterns, and also the facilities it has available for the storage of food. The sleeping arrangements for the family and the sleeping patterns of each member are directly related to insufficient rest, and the resultant physical or emotional health problems.

The importance of the environment and its associated factors is taking on new significance today in relation to health and health problems. The home, although not an intact microcosm of society, nevertheless has many of the same environmental characteristics in relation to health. The amount of living space, the type of toilet facilities, the sources and amount of water available, and the presence of flies, rodents, and accident hazards are directly related to mental disorders, infectious diseases, food poisoning, rat bites, accidents, and lead poisoning.

The medical history of each family member and the current illnesses, including treatments and medications, are important items in the definition of health problems. The medical history not only points out past health problems but also indicates specific areas in which disease prevention and health promotion are necessary. The presence of acute or chronic illness in one family member is a key indicator to possible family health problems, as illness always has some effect on the equilibrium of the family and its ability to carry out its functions. Emotional, social, and physical health problems which follow a family pattern are also discernible from the health history.

As discussed earlier, the base-line information necessary for the community health nurse to have about a family may be similar to that which is necessary for other professionals. However, the uniqueness of each profession lies in the kinds of questions each asks about similar data. In the following discussion the steps in the analysis of health-related data for the identification of family nursing needs are discussed, and some of the questions to be asked by the community health nurse are highlighted.

The steps in the analysis of the data directly related to health problems in the identification of nursing needs are to determine:

1. The relationship of the items to each other.
2. The relationship of the items to the health of the individuals.
3. The relationship of the individual's health problems to the family as a whole.
4. The final determination of family health problems or potential problems.
5. The contribution of nursing to the solution of the health problems.
6. The statement of family nursing needs.

Relationship of the Items to Each Other

As has been pointed out, each item gives some clues about the possibility of the presence of family health problems. However, it is only when the items are analyzed in relation to each other that the basis for a beginning understanding of health disequilibrium in the family becomes evident.

Questions the community health nurse asks to help clarify these relationships might be: What does the demographic data about age, sex, and so forth have to do with the accident hazards? What is the relationship, if any, of the medical history to the sleeping arrangements or the living space? How do the facilities for the storage of food affect the eating patterns? Are the current treatments and medications consistent with the current illnesses?

Relationship of the Items to the Health of the Individuals

After the effect of the individual items upon each other has been ascertained, then the data are analyzed to determine the impact of these relationships on the health of the individuals in the family.

Suggested questions to be asked include: What effect does the eating pattern have on the family member with diabetes or one who is obese? What is the relationship of the sleeping patterns to the emotional development of the individual? What is the relationship of the pattern of family illness to the age and sex of the children? Answers to these and similar questions will help to clarify the health problems of the individual members.

Relation of the Individual's Health Problems to the Family as a Whole

An exploration of the effect of the health problems of the individuals on the family as a whole makes it possible at this stage to determine some tentative family health problems. The analysis of the data will be clarified by such questions as: What family health problems are triggered because of the use of drugs by the teen-age son or daughter? Does the aged parent contribute to or impair the family equilibrium? What is the effect of the sleeping habits of the individual on the family sleeping arrangements and sleep patterns? A statement of tentative family health problems will ensue from this analysis.

Determination of Family Health Problems or Potential Problems

The tentative family health problems are further clarified, verified, or rejected, and new ones added by an analysis of their relationship with the other base-line information. As stated previously, all the base-line information is characterized by its interrelatedness and cannot be looked at in isolation, although some is more pertinent to one of the steps in the nursing process than to another. Through the analysis with the other base-line information the factors which contribute to the health problems will become evident, and other ones may come to light. For example, lack of finances or of health knowledge may be a contributing factor to the poor eating habits and resultant nutritional problems. Or the role assignments and relationships may be directly related to emotional family health problems not identified earlier. Questions pertaining to family health practices may help to clarify the source of a health problem, thus making it more amenable to solution. From an analysis of the interrelatedness of the base-line information to the tentative family health problems comes the final statement of family health problems.

Contribution of Nursing to the Solution of Family Health Problems

As discussed earlier, a nursing need is the contribution nursing can make to the solution of a health problem. Therefore, the family health problems, real or potential, are the framework within which family nursing needs are identified.

What is the contribution nursing can make to the solution of the family health problems? The community health nurse must examine this question very critically to determine the specific nursing contribution for each health problem. In the solution of some problems there is a major contribution nursing can make, while in the solution of others nursing's contribution is negligible. For example, there is a fairly direct relationship between the alleviation of the health problems associated with the maternity cycle and the contribution of nursing in this area. On the other hand, the contribution of nursing to the health problems of dental care is less clear.

Statement of Family Nursing Needs

The final step in the analysis is the determination by the community health nurse of family nursing needs which she should do something about. In this crucial step she must look at the total base-line information for help in making judgments about the ability of the family to cope with its health problems. How the family has managed with past problems, the sources of help available to them, the strength of the family as a group, and the health behaviors which need to be strengthened, those which need to be changed, and those which should be left alone are some of the factors she must weigh in this final step of the analysis. A family member, a neighbor, or other health professional may be adequately meeting some of the nursing needs; thus, these are the needs which she should leave alone.

It is from this kind of analysis that the community health nurse will make the final determination and statements of the family nursing needs. From these statements the nursing actions to meet the needs will be planned.

In this chapter the base-line information about the family has been categorized in relation to the items most directly related to defining family health problems and to planning and implementing the family nursing care plan. Clues to be obtained in relation to each item were discussed briefly.

The steps in the analysis of the data to determine family nursing needs were outlined. A nursing need was defined as the contribution of nursing to the solution of a health problem. In the seventies, a time of increasingly sophisticated technology, rapidly changing health delivery systems, expanding health teams, and strong societal forces, it is imperative that the community health nurse clearly understand her contribution to the health of families in order to make sound professional judgments about their nursing needs.

REFERENCES

DeYoung, C. Nursing's contribution in family crisis treatment. Nurs. Outlook, 16:60-62, February 1968.

Godde, W. The Sociology of the Family—Horizons in Family Theory. In Merton, R., Broom, L., and Cottrell, L., Jr., eds., Sociology Today: Problems and Prospects. New York, Harper and Row, 1965, Ch. 7, 178-196.

Helvie, C., Hill, A., and Bambino, C. The setting and nursing practice, Part II. Nurs. Outlook, 16:35-38, September 1968.

Hill, R., and Hansen, D. The identification of conceptual frameworks utilized in family study. Marriage and Family Living, 22:299-311, November 1960.

Kluckholm, R. Family diagnosis. Social Casework, 39:63-72, February-March 1958.

Nye, I., and Berardo, F. Emerging Conceptual Frameworks in Family Analysis. New York, The Macmillan Company, 1966.

Schwartz, D., Henley, B., and Leitz, L. The Elderly Ambulatory Patient: Nursing and Psychosocial Needs. New York, The Macmillan Company, 1964.

Wald, F., and Leonard, R. Towards development of nursing practice theory. Nurs. Res., 13:309-313, Fall 1964.

CHAPTER 8

Developing the Family Nursing Care Plan

The nursing needs of families that have been identified by the community health nurse form the basis for the development of a nursing care plan. The nursing care plan is the blueprint which gives direction to the nursing intervention that ensues. It consists of the specific nursing goals for the family and the specific nursing action needed to reach the goals. The importance of the mutual dependence of the goals and the actions must not be underestimated. The clear statement of the goals for nursing intervention in the family makes purposive nursing activity possible. In other words, if the nursing goals are not clear, it really does not make much difference what activities the nurse performs because she does not know where she is going anyway. It is similar to a person who wants to go on a trip but does not know where he wants to go, so he takes the first means of transportation that is available. It will not make any difference what means of transportation he selects, as he does not know where he is going anyway. The nursing action to meet the goals also must be clearly stated; otherwise, the nursing activity may or may not be directed to the goals and becomes purposeless. There may be several nursing actions that can be taken, just as there may be many means of transportation for someone going on a trip, but the selection of activities must be clearly stated and be goal-directed. The statements of nursing goals and of nursing action are dependent upon an accurate identification of nursing needs. If these are not identified accurately, the resultant nursing goals and actions will have limited results and could have an adverse effect on the family in its movement toward a high level of well-being. The community health nurse, because of her education and experience, must assume the responsibility and the concomitant accountability for identifying the nursing needs of families and for developing the nursing care plan based on those needs.

The nursing needs of the family as a whole are the central focus, although each family member has an effect and is affected by the plan which evolves. Much of the nursing intervention may be directed at one individual, but the overall purpose is to improve the functioning of the family as a unit. Working with the individuals is one way this purpose can be achieved. The relationships of the individual to the total health of the family has some of the same elements that are found in the relationship of the family to the total health of the community. Just as the health of the family is reflected in the health of the community, the health of the individual is reflected in the health of the family.

In determining the nursing care plan some of the basic assumptions about the practice of community health nursing must be kept in mind. One of these is that the family has the right and responsibility to make its own decisions. Another is that the community health nurse works with the family in determining its health problems, in developing the plan of action, and in evaluating the outcomes. These assumptions make it clear that the active involvement of the family with the community health nurse, in mutually identifying its needs and planning the nursing action, is essential in community health nursing practice. People themselves are the ones who make their own problems and they also have the ability to solve them. To do this they must have correct and adequate information to make sound decisions. They also must be involved early in the decision-making process and in any plans which are developed. We all know of many laudable plans which have been developed but have died an early death because the people who were to be affected most by the plans were not consulted or involved as they were being developed. The early involvement of the family in the decision-making process is as applicable for the community health nurse as she works with her families as it is in all other endeavors in the life of the people. Unless the community health nurse really believes in the ability of people to solve their own problems, she will be ineffective in her nursing practice with families.

Community health nursing has a long history of working with families and with lay persons in developing nursing services. One of its basic assumptions is that people in the community are indispensable in all phases of the community health nursing program. Their experiences and commitment to this assumption are particularly pertinent at the present time, with the demands by consumers of all kinds for control of the services they receive. These demands by the consumers are having a profound effect on professional workers in all areas. The education and experience of professional persons, for the most part, have not prepared them to participate with the consumers as colleagues in the decision-making process about the kind and quality of professional services to be rendered. As a result, no precedents have been established that can be used as guidelines, and there is much confusion by consumers and professionals alike about who has what responsibility and authority. Reaction on the part of the professional workers has been varied. Some have withdrawn completely and ignored the demands, an action which has tended to increase the tension from all sides. Others have abdicated their professional responsibility, with the consumer making all of the decisions, an action which also tended to increase the tension and conflict. Others, similar to the long tradition of community health nursing in working with lay persons, are developing a partnership with consumer groups in which the knowledge of the professional and the needs of the consumer are shared, and mutually acceptable decisions are made about the kind and quality of services to be offered.

There is no doubt about the fact that a new era of consumer participation is in the offing which will markedly change the traditional patterns of providing services of all kinds to people. Out of this, either new and more relevant roles for the existing professions must emerge, or new professions will evolve to meet the demands.

Nursing practice, as was discussed in Chapter 5, has adhered closely to the medical model in which all information about the patient is directed to the physician, who in turn makes the decisions regarding the services that should be rendered. With this model the professional worker, especially the physician, has more information about the patient than the patient, who is to receive the services, has about himself. This model, which does not include involvement of people in making their own decisions, is no longer relevant for the individual, the family, or the community.

The family and its needs are the focus of the community health nurse. The family must make its own decisions about the nursing services that it needs, wants, and will use. However, it cannot make these decisions and understand the implications of alternate choices unless it has adequate and correct information. The family model, in which all the information about the family is directed to the family so that it may make sound decisions about the services it receives, is the operating model for the community health nurse. The family provides the nurse with information about the family situation, and the nurse provides the family with professional knowledge and information. Each in this sense is the expert in his respective role. This information is then pooled and mutual decisions reached about the services to be rendered. This kind of collaborative relationship strengthens the role of the community health nurse—rather than diminishing it, as some nurses fear—by forcing her to clearly identify the contribution nursing can make and interpreting this to the family. The contributions, or goals, of nursing differ from those of other disciplines, although they may have similar roles and functions. Herein lies the uniqueness of nursing!

As was discussed in the previous chapter, some of the base-line information needed about a family is more pertinent in developing the nursing plan of care and must be considered in this phase of the nursing process. These items are shown in Table 1.

TABLE 1

**Items directly related to developing the family
nursing care plan**

Education
Ethnic and religious practices
Health knowledge
Health practices

Health problems as seen by family
Health problems as seen by nurse
Income and expenses
Medical and dental care
Method of payment for medical and dental
    care
Patterns of decision making
Relationship of members to each other
Type of neighborhood
Use of leisure

The knowledge, judgment, and sensitivity of the community health nurse is of paramount importance in the value and use of this information in the development of the nursing care plan.

The steps in the process of its development include:

1. Determining the relationship of the nursing need to other needs in the family.
2. Establishing the priority of nursing need.
3. Establishing the nursing goals.
4. Determining the nursing action to meet the goals.

Evaluation is inherent in each of these steps.

The Relationship of Nursing Needs to Other Family Needs

Families, similar to communities, have multiple needs. These cover many areas and include social, religious, cultural, economic, recreation, health, employment, housing, education, and nursing needs to name a few. These needs are constantly vying for attention, with both the internal and external forces operating in the family at any one time setting the stage for this drama.

The nursing needs must be looked at in relation to the other needs of the family. Nursing and health may be high on the priority list and occupy center stage, or it may be at the bottom of the list and not even be waiting in the wings. However, no one category of need has the same priority all the time; either because the need has been met for the time being or because other events have occurred, such as illness in the breadwinner, making a reshuffling of priorities necessary. In developing the nursing care plan the community health nurse has to keep these facts in mind, and determine the relationship of the nursing needs to the other needs in the family. It may be that the nursing needs cannot be met until a job is found for the husband, or that before anything can be done about improving the nutritional status of the family, the marital problems have to be resolved. The value system of the family, which is a powerful determinant of its behavior, is a decisive factor to be considered in determining the hierarchy of needs and the relation of nursing to this hierarchy.

Priority of Nursing Needs

The nursing needs, in turn, have their own priority which must be established before the nursing action can be planned. Matching the nursing needs with the pertinent base-line information which was collected about the family, and with the available resources in the family and the community, will help determine the relative importance of each need and how best to meet it. Part of this process includes a determination of the strengths and weaknesses in a family. Families are generally much more aware of their weaknesses than of their strengths. Invariably, however, the strengths far outweigh the weaknesses, and it behooves the community health nurse to ascertain and exploit the strengths the family has. They also have some potential strengths which may have been lying dormant because there had been no opportunity available for their use. This knowledge plus the base-line information collected relating to how the family has managed before in similar situations, or when faced with a stressful or crisis situation, will enable the community health nurse to make a judgment about the family's ability to cope with its health problems and nursing needs.

The relative importance of each nursing need and the plan to meet it also depend upon the relationship of the nursing needs to other pertinent information about the family. The educational level and the coping ability of the family, but also give some idea about the needs will have a direct bearing on the amount of information to include in the nursing plan, and the method of teaching to be used. The relationships within the family not only help to clarify further the coping ability of the family, but also give some ideas about the kind of support and mutual help that is available.

One of the purposes for nursing intervention in the family is to increase its knowledge about health and to help change some of its health practices. The nursing needs are directly related to these areas, and the relationship between health knowledge and health practices the coping ability of the family, but also give some ideas about the family regarding health may have to be the first step in nursing intervention before any other results can be obtained. Health practices, although not necessarily related to health knowledge can be influenced by a greater awareness of current family health practices and provide an opportunity to explore alternative choices. Health knowledge and practices are also closely allied to the educational level of the family and how it gets information about health. The amount of information one obtains through reading tends to get larger as the educational level increases. Persons who utilize televison and the radio as their main sources of information tend to be less well-informed than the "readers." The ethnic heritage and religious background of a family has a tremendous influence on its health practices. The kind of food, how it is cooked, and when it is eaten are related to the ethnic and cultural heritage as well as to religious beliefs and customs. Other practices, such as the role of women, decision making, discipline, and permissible social behavior, are related to both the cultural and religious beliefs. These family practices in turn influence the priority that will be given to the nursing needs. The most important nursing need may be given a low priority by the family because it is in direct conflict to the cultural and religious practices.

There is no one pattern that determines what individuals or families perceive as their health problems and needs. Vickers[1] mentions that much depends upon the degree to which the individual seeks either to preserve an internal or external relation which he needs or thinks he needs, or to escape threats to a relation which will strain it beyond repair. The first he describes as goal-seeking—the successful completion of a goal in which the individual then decides whether the goal was worth seeking. The latter he defines as threat-avoiding—the successful avoidance of a threat so that the individual never has the opportunity of experiencing it and never knows if it was worth avoiding. These two approaches of goal-seeking or threat-avoiding are strong forces operating in a family when it attempts to determine its health problems. The health problems as seen by the family may be based on knowledge and sound logic, or they may be the result of long-standing practices and superstitions which have been passed down from generation to generation. The community health nurse must understand what the family believes its health problems to be and the basis for its belief. The priority of nursing

---

[1] Vickers, G. What sets the goals in public health? *New Eng. J. Med.*, 258:589-596, March 1958.

needs will be directly affected by the intensity with which family problems are perceived.

The health problems as seen by the family may be different from those seen by the nurse. This is not unique to community health nursing, as there is always a gap between the knowledge and understandings professional workers have about health and those held by the consumers. However, in establishing the priority of nursing needs the community health nurse must recognize that this gap may exist and work with the family to resolve the differences. By keeping the family and its health problems as the major reason for her services, the nurse narrows the gaps in perception and clarifies the priority of nursing needs. The improvement of the overall health status of the community is the ultimate aim of community health nursing, with the family as the vehicle through which this is accomplished. Therefore, the nursing services provided by the community health nurse are directly related to the health problems and priorities which have been established by the community. The priority of nursing needs in the family will not necessarily be the same as the priorities of the larger community. However, the nursing needs will be influenced by the priorities and by the accepted behaviors which are sanctioned by the community.

As can be seen by the foregoing discussion, the nursing needs of a family are only one small part of the whole constellation of family needs. In each family the priority of needs will depend upon many factors which influence the place of health in the hierarchy of needs. Similarly, the identified nursing needs will also have a priority of their own and will be based upon many of the same factors that determine the priority of other needs in the family.

Establishing Nursing Goals

The development of the nursing care plan can begin to take shape after the priority of nursing needs has been established. This is a joint venture, with the nurse and the family working closely together in all the phases. The choice of which individual or individuals in the family will participate is dependent upon the family decision-making pattern and how final decisions are made.

The plan, even though it is developed jointly with the nurse and the family, must be one that will be adhered to by the family. It may have been developed in a time of crisis, and when the crisis no longer seems imminent the plan may be abandoned. Or, too high a degree of commitment of the family over a long period of time may be required, which it is not ready to accept and carry through. The acceptability of the plan in the neighborhood must also be taken into consideration. It must be congruent with the sanctions imposed by the neighborhood if it is to be adhered to. For example, if the plan involves a change in the sleeping patterns of the family that is in conflict with those of the neighborhood, the value of this for the family should be weighed against the misunderstanding and disapproval of the neighborhood.

The effect of the plan on the family as a whole is another consideration. What changes in the assigned roles of each individual are necessary, and will this have a positive or negative influence? If because of the illness of the mother, a 14-year-old daughter has to assume the homemaking responsibilities, what effect will this have on the daughter and on the family? On the other hand, one of the nursing goals may be to strengthen the family by more appropriate role assignments; thus, the role changes may be disruptive at first, but the long-range outcomes will be of value to the family as a unit.

Are the necessary resources available in the neighborhood to carry out the plan, and what is the reaction of the people to their use? As was discussed in the previous chapter, adequate facilities may be available in a community, but they may not be used because of misconceptions by the people about the services or because they are inaccessible due to lack of transportation. If the resources are not available in the neighborhood, where can they be found? Is transportation available, and how can it be arranged? Long waiting lists for admission to hospitals and other health care facilities are not unusual today. How does this affect the nursing care plan? What are the alternatives to being at the bottom of a long waiting list?

The financial cost to the family, and what this means to the total budget is a major consideration. The costs and charges of nursing visits from home health agencies, as with all other health services, are soaring. Even though the American people have agreed that health is the right of each individual citizen, and legislation has been passed to help to realize this ideal, the quality of health care received by individuals is still closely related to their ability to pay for it.

The source of medical care for the family will influence the development of the nursing care plan. The method of payment for medical care has some bearing on the source of care. If the local druggist is the source of much of the medical information, with the hospital emergency room as a last resort, how a plan which includes regular visits to a physician will be adhered to by the family must be considered.

One of the overall purposes of community health nursing is to help families help themselves. The movement of a family from dependency to independence is inherent in this purpose and should be reflected in the nursing care plan. In this movement, however, it should be kept in mind that contrary to popular thought, independence is not always a virtue and dependency is not always a vice. It may be as important to help a person to be dependent as to be independent. The autonomous nuclear family of today is much more dependent upon extrafamilial institutions and other resources than ever before. In order to fulfill its functions as a family it must know what facilities are available and how to use them. In this sense they may have to learn that some dependence is essential in order for optimal family functioning. By the same token, the highly independent individual who has had a myocardial infarction must learn to have a degree of dependence if he wishes to live out his normal life span.

The heart of the nursing care plan is transposing the nursing needs into realizable goals. This, as in all the other phases, is a joint venture which involves both the family and the nurse, with the family situation and its needs as the axis around which the nursing goals are defined. Family nursing goals give direction to the ensuing nursing actions and provide criteria for evaluating the outcomes. The goals are the road or path which the community health nurse travels in helping families solve their health problems to enable them to function at their highest possible level. The level of family functioning is one indicator of its health status.

The statement of nursing goals should indicate the health behaviors or observable facts in the family's ability to promote and maintain health and to prevent disease. The family and what it can do, rather than the nurse and what she does, is the main focus of the stated goals. For example, a goal which states, "To increase the family's understanding of budgeting," gives some idea about what the nurse will do, but does not indicate in any way what the family will be able to do. The same goal stated in behavioral terms might be "Husband and wife plan budget together," or "The budget is made out weekly," or "Each family member who contributes to the income participates in decisions about the budget." In these statements the emphasis is on the expected behavior from the family because of the nursing contribution. The outcomes can be evaluated through observation of changes in family behavior.

It is highly unlikely that the nursing needs of any family would ever result in only one nursing goal. Instead, they are more apt to fall into categories of goals. As the main focus of the community health nurse is on family health promotion, health maintenance, and disease prevention, the nursing goals can be categorized under these same headings. The completed statements will give a composite picture of the nursing goals for the family and will highlight the category in which there seems to be the greatest emphasis. Thus, it becomes possible to capture quickly the relation of one category to the other, to determine the short- and long-range goals, and to identify clearly the nursing action necessary to reach the goals. At the same time it provides the opportunity to pinpoint the highest priority of nursing goals and the timing of nursing action.

If the community health nurse is to categorize nursing goals under the headings of health promotion, health maintenance, and disease prevention, she must be clear about the nursing contribution in each of these categories. The nursing contribution can be defined as follows:

1. *Health promotion:* to increase the level of understanding and the expectations of health for the family. This may include changing or modifying health practices, increasing health knowledge, and developing understanding of normal growth and development.

2. *Health maintenance:* to maintain the family as a group in handling its health problems. This may include therapeutic nursing services, help in time of crisis, such as illness, birth, or hospitalization, and coordination of health and nursing services.

3. *Disease prevention:* to maintain and increase the level of immunization in the family to prevent the occurrence or recurrence of disease or illness. Level of immunization includes developing resistance to the social, emotional, and biologic forces which precipitate disease or illness. This encompasses such things as increasing knowledge about preventive measures in relation to specific diseases, such as special diets, breast self-examination, and vaccines; furthering understanding of the connection of the interpersonal relationships in the family with disease occurrence; and stimulating the family to participate in health screening and immunization programs.

With these definitions in mind the community health nurse can then transpose the nursing needs into realizable nursing goals under one of these categories. Some statements of goals related to the expected family behavior under each of these headings might be:

Health Promotion

All family members have adequate sleeping arrangements.

The family eats at least one meal together each day.

Expectations of the children's behavior are appropriate to their age and sex.

Positive health knowledge is shared with friends and neighbors.

Health Maintenance

All family members participate in some way in caring for a sick member.

The family actively seeks help in time of crisis.

The family uses community health resources appropriately.

Each family member sees a physician for periodic checkups.

Disease Prevention

The diabetic diet is consistently carried out without disruption of family food patterns.

No family member is a scapegoat.

Each child has the necessary immunizations and boosters.

In determining which of the goals have the highest priority, the relationship of health promotion, health maintenance, and prevention of disease should be assessed very critically to determine the long-range impact on the family. For example, if most of the nursing goals are primarily in the area of therapeutic nursing services, what will happen to the family in the future if prevention and health promotion are neglected today? In determining the priority of nursing goals, the immediate and long-range outcomes for the family must not be forgotten. In some situations the long-range outcomes are more important and should have high priority, even if this should be more disrupting to the immediate situation. The knowledge, skill, and judgment of the community health nurse is of prime importance in this deliberation.

After the priority of nursing goals has been established, the next step in the process is to determine short-term goals which should be developed to facilitate movement toward the larger goals. The short-term goals give immediate direction for the nursing action, make it possible to have periodic evaluation of the nursing contribution and to evaluate the long-term goal and restate it if necessary. An example under each of the categories will illustrate the selection of short-term goals.

One of the health promotion goals was, "The family eats at least one meal together each day." To achieve this may require completely changing family eating patterns, changing the family's feelings about food, finding different ways of buying and cooking food, finding different food storage procedures, and changing the amount of money allocated for food. Each of these can be stated as expected family behaviors, and the outcomes can be observed and evaluated. For instance, let us assume that one of the stated short-term goals is, "The amount of money allotted for food is increased by 10 percent." By the time this goal is accomplished and evaluated, it is found that one of the family members has a new job in which he works from 4:00 P.M. to 12:00 midnight for 5 days per week. Immediately it becomes obvious that the long-range goal of the family eating at least one meal together each day cannot be achieved. As a result it is evaluated and restated as, "The family eats at least one meal together on weekends," or "Family members whose working hours permit eat at least one meal together each day." Without the short-range goal with its built-in evaluation, the longer goal might not have been changed.

One of the health maintenance goals stated, "All family members participate in some way in caring for the sick member." This may require teaching someone to give nursing care between the visits of the nurse, planning special foods, entertaining the sick member, relieving the caretaker so he or she may have recreation, changing the sleeping arrangements, keeping a supply of fresh linen on hand, and reallocating the budget items to meet extra expenses incurred by the sickness. In this situation a short-term goal may be, "The mother gives therapeutic nursing care between visits of the nurse." When this goal is reached, the evaluation indicates that the larger goal is still realistic and reachable, and progress toward reaching it is continued.

An example of a goal under Disease Prevention was stated, "Each child has the necessary immunizations and boosters." Because of the family situation, it may be determined that this goal in itself is a short-range goal. The family already understands the value of immunizations, and it is only necessary to remind it of the time when they are due, to keep them informed of new developments, and at intervals to reinterpret their value.

As can be seen, there are many aspects to consider in establishing the nursing goals. The key to making the goals have meaning is to state them in behavioral terms which can be evaluated. Three questions can be asked in evaluating the clarity of the statements of nursing goals. These are:

1. Are the goals acceptable to the family?
2. Is it clear where the family is going?
3. Can we tell when they get there?

If the answer is "yes" to all of these, then the nursing action to meet the goals can be determined.

Determining Nursing Action

Once again it must be stressed that in actuality it is very difficult to separate nursing action from nursing goals, as they are often developed simultaneously. However, as has been mentioned many times, we believe that by breaking the various steps into small component parts the total nursing process becomes clearer and more easily understood.

The nursing actions necessary to carry out the nursing goals are easily discernible when the expected behaviors are clear. The category of the goal also helps to highlight the nursing action. The goals and nursing action to achieve them must be mutually agreed upon by the family and the nurse. The nurse has the responsibility of providing the family with sufficient and accurate information upon which it can base its decisions about what it wants to do and what it can do. The nurse must help the family to look at alternative choices and at their possible effects on the solution of the family health problem. The final decision about what nursing actions are acceptable rests with the family. As mentioned earlier, one of the basic assumptions of community health nursing practice is the right and responsibility of the family to make its own decisions. The importance of this assumption in this stage of the development of the nursing care plan cannot be emphasized enough. It is necessary that the nurse make sure that the family has all the available information and that it clearly understands the alternative choices. This is solely the responsibility of the nurse, but she must also support the family in whatever decisions it makes. For example, one of the nursing goals with resultant nursing action might be for the teen-age son with diabetes to be advised to give himself his own insulin, whereupon he refuses to accept this responsibility. The nurse should give him accurate and adequate information about the alternative choices to administering his own insulin and their consequences to him in the future as well as the present. The final choice rests with him, and the community health nurse supports his decision and works with him in planning the nursing actions which are appropriate to the decision he made.

The overall functions of the community health nurse in the family include direct nursing care, health teaching, referral, health counseling, anticipatory guidance, planning, collaboration, coordination, and health advocacy. Some of these are independent functions and some are dependent. The degree of independence and dependence is determined by each family situation. Bergman[2] has defined three levels of nursing activities by which she differentiates the independent and dependent functions of the community health nurse. They are:

1. *Assisting activities:* these facilitate the work initiated by another person who is responsible for the outcome. Examples are the nurse assisting a physician with a physical examination, or administering medications ordered by the physician.
2. *Complementing activities:* these are initiated by another person, but the nurse adds a specific nursing dimension for which she has responsibility. Examples are teaching a person with diabetes how to plan his diet which has been ordered by the physician, or planning and arranging for school health examinations.
3. *Initiating activities:* the need is recognized by the nurse who initiates action. Examples would be identifying nursing needs and planning the necessary nursing action to alleviate the need, i.e., helping the family cope with its health problems; or planning and conducting nutrition classes for obese teenagers.

The nursing action to carry out the functions are many and varied. The same holds true in the choices of nursing action to meet the nursing goals of a family. Because of this there are limitless opportunities for creative nursing actions which will enhance the family's ability to solve its own health problems. The nursing goals give direction to the type of nursing action, such as teaching, giving direct nursing care, anticipatory guidance, and so forth. However, the specific action and how it is carried out depends upon the creativity of the nurse as she works with the family in presenting alternative choices. To illustrate, one of the goals under health maintenance was, "The mother gives therapeutic nursing care between the visits of the nurse." The goal requires that the nursing action be geared toward

[2] Bergman, R. L. Public health nursing functions: Assisting, complementing, initiating. *Nurs. Outlook,* 14:42-43, July 1966.

teaching the mother to give the necessary care. However, how and what is taught will vary widely, depending upon the individual situation and what is acceptable to the mother and the family. This is where the creative potential of the nurse can come into full play.

The final consideration in planning the nursing actions is the estimated number of community health nurse contacts which will be necessary. How many home visits should be planned? Will attendance at group meetings, for example, parents' classes or the local Association for Retarded Children, alter the number of home visits? What kinds of information can be transmitted by the telephone? How many contacts with other professional and nonprofessional workers on behalf of the family will be necessary? If it is impractical or impossible to provide the number of estimated contacts, what are the alternatives and what will be the effect on the solution of the family health problems? Are the estimated number and kind of visits consistent with the policies governing the community health nursing program, or shall an exception be made for this family? Perhaps all the policies need to be reevaluated and changes made to meet the demands of consumers for more relevant services.

Evaluation of the nursing actions are continuous and ongoing. When changes occur in the family situation or in either the long- or short-range nursing goals, appropriate changes must be made in the nursing actions to coincide with the changed situations.

The component parts in the development of a nursing care plan have been discussed in this chapter. The identified nursing needs, which have been defined as the contribution nursing can make to the solution of a health problem, were the framework upon which the nursing goals and resultant nursing actions were built. Each step in the process of the development of the plan was discussed as it was affected by the family and it effected the family. The steps were: determining the relationship of the nursing needs to other needs in the family; establishing priority of nursing needs; establishing the nursing goals; and determining the nursing action to meet the goals. The implementation and evaluation of the plan are the subjects of the next chapter.

REFERENCES

Buckles, J., Cashar, L., and Olson, L. Learning purposeful nursing intervention. Amer. J. Nurs., 68:2578-2580, December 1968.

Bergman, R. L. Public health nursing functions: Assisting, complementing, initiating. Nurs. Outlook, 14:42-44, July 1966.

Fox, D. J. A proposed model for identifying research areas in nursing. Nurs. Res., 13:29-36, Winter 1964.

Griffiths, E. I. A rational approach to patient service review. Nurs. Outlook, 17:49-51, April 1969.

Harris, F. L. Who needs written care plans anyway? Amer. J. Nurs., 70:2136-2138, October 1970.

Helvie, C., Hill, A., and Bambino, C. The setting and nursing practice, Part II. Nurs. Outlook, 16:35-38, September 1968.

Levine, M. E. Adaptation and assessment. A rationale for nursing intervention. Amer. J. Nurs., 66:2450-2453, November 1966.

National Commission of Community Health Services. Health Is a Community Affair. Cambridge, Massachusetts, Harvard University Press, 1967.

Otto, H. A. Developing Family Strengths and Potential. In Otto, H., and Mann, J., eds., Ways of Growth. New York, Grossman Publishers, 1968, Ch. 8, pp. 77-85.

Palisin, H. E. Nursing care plans are a snare and a delusion. Amer. J. Nurs., 71:63-66, January 1971.

Smith, D. M. Writing objectives as a nursing practice skill. Amer. J. Nurs., 71:319-420, February 1971.

Stewart, R., and Graham, J. Evaluation tools in public health nursing. Nurs. Outlook, 16:50-51, March 1968.

Vickers, G. What sets the goals in public health? New. Eng. J. Med., 258:589-596, March 1958.

Webber, M. The Prospects for Policies Planning. In Duhl, L. J., ed., The Urban Condition, New York, Simon and Schuster, 1969, Ch. 25, pp. 319-330.

CHAPTER 9

Implementing and Evaluating the Family Nursing Plan

None of the steps in the nursing process can be carried out as discrete, separate entities. At any one time there is much overlapping, with each step dependent upon and interchangeable with the other steps. This overlapping, dependency, and interchangeability is particularly evident in the planning and implementing phases, as implementation is inherent in developing any kind of plan. However, in order to understand more clearly the many facets involved in implementing the family nursing care plan, we have attempted to separate the two steps—but always lurking in the back of our minds are the pitfalls of this approach.

The nursing actions that will move the family toward reaching the nursing goals have been identified mutually by the family and the community health nurse. The nurse has the responsibility for mobilizing all the available resources in implementing the actions. What parts of the plan must the nurse carry out herself, and what parts can be done by others? In answering this question she takes into consideration the roles and functions of other professional and nonprofessional workers, and their effect on the particular family and its health problems. The nursing goals for a family are different than the goals of other health professionals, but many of the functions of other workers are similar to those of nurses. In fact, the functions of all health workers have many similarities, with much overlapping and duplication. In addition, the roles and relationships of each health worker are very fluid and are constantly being revised. The degree of this similarity in function and fluidity of roles becomes strikingly evident when the family and its health problems are the focus of care. Because of this some of the nursing goals of families can be met by other professionals, such as a physician, a social worker, or an occupational therapist. Similarly, some of the goals of these workers can be met by the actions of the nurse. Families also provide a wide variety of health care for their members. The actions of the family members are vitally important in the movement of the family toward a high level of well-being.

Increasingly, the multidiscipline health team providing comprehensive health services will become the pattern of health delivery for the majority of people. In these situations today, community health nurses are collaborating as full-fledged team members with other health professionals, and a peer group collegiality is developing. With the health problems of the patient and his family as the hub around which the team operates, the contribution of each team member is becoming more clearly defined for himself and for others. It is being cogently demonstrated that through this kind of approach new roles and functions emerge; at the same time the goals and contributions of each professional becomes more important and necessary.

The responsibilities the community health nurse has in implementing the nursing care plan include:

1. Making decisions about carrying out the plan.
2. Providing nursing services.
3. Revising the nursing care plan.
4. Making referrals and collaborating with others in behalf of the family.
5. Coordinating the nursing and health services to the family.
6. Participating in continuing professional development.

Some of the base-line information collected about the family has more relevance in this step of the nursing process than in the other steps. The information is shown in Table 1. The community health nurse should be constantly alert to the relationship of these items to each other and to the total family situation as she implements the nursing care plan.

TABLE 1

Items directly related to implementing the family
nursing care plan

Availability and accessibility of health
facilities
Expectations of services of community
health nurse
Participation in community activities
Past experience with health professionals
Relationship of family to larger community
Role assignment
Role model of parents
Sources of help used by family
Transportation facilities
Use of community agencies
Value system

Making Decisions About Carrying Out the Plan

The resourcefulness and creativity of the community health nurse play an important part in how she uses the clues she garners from the available information as she moves into the decision-making phase of implementation. Data about the role model of the parents and the role assignments of family members help to determine what aspect of the plan can be carried out by the family itself, and the amount of support and continuous participation that can be expected. The sources of help the family have used before should be looked at, and their pertinence to the present situation ascertained.

Perhaps the sources are still available and accessible to the family. At the same time there may be persons to whom the family members turn for guidance and whose opinions have a significant effect on the family. These persons are referred to as the *significant others* and are often overlooked by professional workers. As the nuclear family becomes more and more specialized, and as other family relatives become more dispersed, significant others, such as close friends, will play an ever-increasing role as sources of help and emotional support for families. Neighbors also have a bearing on how the plan may be implemented, although the role of neighbors, particularly in the impersonal environment of large urban areas, is changing as rapidly as every other facet of society.

The values of the family and the importance they place on health also influences how the plan will be carried out. This is a particularly difficult area for the community health nurse, as many times she finds her values in direct conflict with the values of the family. The conflict may be centered around moral and religious beliefs, such as those concerning illegitimacy and abortion. Cultural differences, such as the use of practices that seem to be opposite to present-day scientific principles, often evoke conflict. Others, such as how the family spends its money, how it disciplines its children, and the cleanliness of the house, are less obvious value-conflict producers, but can exert tremendous pressures when they are in opposition to strong beliefs held by the nurse. Working with families who have value systems different from her own does not mean that the nurse gives up her own beliefs and embraces those of the family. It does mean, however, that she recognizes the differences and guards against imposing her own values on families as she helps them to solve their own health problems within their own situation. This is consistent with one of the basic assumptions of community health nursing practice, that the family has the right and responsibility to make its own decisions.

The family is the patient of the community health nurse, and she must consider the effect that the presence of an ill member will have on the others in the family; and how the ill member affects the ability of the family to function as a group. In spite of some current thinking to the contrary, the family may not be the best setting for the ill member, and a more appropriate facility may have to be found. If he is to remain at home, the length of time the family can be expected to care for him and the kind of help it will need are factors to keep in mind.

The available health resources and facilities and how they can be mobilized will affect how the plan is implemented. On the one hand, there may be a dearth of facilities, and the nurse will have to determine how to get the necessary services. At the other extreme, there may be a plethora of facilities, and the nurse will be confronted with selecting the ones that will best meet the needs of the individual and the family.

Knowledge about the availability of transportation helps the community health nurse in making decisions about the most effective use of community resources. There is no one decision that applies to every family. In some situations it will be more beneficial to the family to have the health worker come into the home to provide the necessary services. At other times maximum benefits at lower cost will be achieved by transporting the individual to a community resource.

Who carries out what part of the plan will also depend upon the past experiences of the family with community health nurses and other health workers. Its past experiences will color the expectations of the amount and kind of nursing services it will expect and accept. This is also true of the services it will accept from other kinds of health workers. The consumer is becoming more and more involved in determining the kind of health care he wants and is demanding that the care he receives be rendered by qualified professionals. The lower income segment of the population, in particular, is demanding that their neighborhood health centers be staffed by full-fledged practitioners. They are rejecting many of the services provided by less well-prepared personnel.

The relationship of the family to the larger community is also considered when deciding who can best carry out the nursing care plan. If the nursing actions are not consistent with current customs and values in the neighborhood, the family may lose face and become alienated from its neighbors. If the usual activities of the family do not include participation in social and health programs in the community, it will be more difficult for it to use the resources which are available.

Providing Nursing Services   The community health nurse weighs all the foregoing factors in making her judgments about who can best provide the nursing services needed by the family and how these services can be implemented. In some instances it may be imperative for the nurse to provide the services herself, whereas in other situations she may supervise others who are providing it. An axiom for her to follow in making her determination is to ask, "What is the least preparation needed to carry out the nursing action?" She must keep in mind that manpower and talent are wasted if persons are providing services that can be done as well or better by persons with less preparation. Concomitantly she must be aware of the danger of assigning tasks that are beyond the training or competence of the person.

If the functions require a high degree of skill or a special type of relationship, the community health nurse may provide all the services herself. She also may give the services herself in order to serve as a role model for others to emulate. In still other cases she may give the services herself in order to demonstrate or to teach someone else how to carry out the functions. On the other hand, she may not provide any of the services herself, but will work with the other workers who are involved. In each instance, however, she still retains responsibility for the quality of nursing care the family receives. In asking herself what is the least preparation needed to carry out the nursing actions, the data may indicate that the nursing needs of the family do not require the special skills of the community health nurse, but can best be met by a registered nurse. On the other hand, it may be that a licensed practical nurse has sufficient competence to carry out the specific nursing action. Or a home health aide, and in some instances a neighborhood aide, may have the requisite skills to meet the nursing needs of the family.

In making determinations about who can best carry out the nursing actions, the family members also play an important role. As mentioned previously, family members provide a great deal of health care and have a reservoir of untapped knowledge and skill in caring for each other which must be understood and utilized to the fullest.

The role of other professionals in carrying out the nursing care plan, which has been discussed previously, should also be exploited in behalf of the family. The community health nurse is responsible for the supervision of all persons providing nursing services to the family. The amount and kind of supervision will vary with each family and with the persons involved in the nursing actions. She serves as a consultant to other professional persons about the nursing needs of families and how they can be met. She also consults with other professionals when their specialized knowledge and skill is required for the family.

Revising the Nursing Care Plan

The community health nurse is constantly searching for new clues which will help her to have a better understanding of the family's health problems and nursing needs. In her search she may discover new relationships among family members, or new health problems unrecognized by the family. She also seeks clues from people outside the immediate family, such as other professional workers who know the family. In families where there are several other professional workers involved, she may initiate a case conference in which all the workers sit down together and share information in order to determine how best the total needs of the family can be met. Relatives can be a source for clues about the family and how they cope with health problems. How and why family members relate to each other and the role each assumes may be particularly puzzling to the nurse. As she observes and gathers clues from relatives about the life style and customs, the interaction pattern of the family members and how they relate to each other can be better understood. Neighbors and significant others are sources of further clues which help the nurse better to understand the family. How the health practices of the family relate to the mores of the neighborhood will increase her understanding about how best to meet the nursing needs of the family.

The family nursing care plan is designed to meet the nursing needs of the family and to help it move toward high-level well-being. The plan to be effective must be based upon information about the family. As new knowledge is obtained, the nursing care plan should be changed accordingly—in other words, the plan is a dynamic, vibrant tool that is responsive to new needs, rather than a static, self-contained instrument. Thus, the interchangeability and interdependence of the steps of the nursing process are demonstrated. Also, the necessity for constant ongoing evaluation of the nursing needs of the family, and of the nursing care plan and its implementation becomes evident. The nursing care plan, and thus its implementation, will change as the family situation changes. Some of the changes, such as when a family member has an acute illness, will pinpoint the need for a change in the plan more dramatically than others, such as the garnering of further information about how the family members relate to each other. In both situations it is conceivable that the nursing goals and nursing action could change, as well as how and by whom the plan is being carried out. The judgments about the significance of the new information and its effect on the nursing goals of the family is the responsibility of the community health nurse.

To meet the changing needs of families today and in the future, it will be necessary to change some of the policies and practices that govern what kind of nursing services are delivered to families and how they are delivered. The working hours of agencies will have to be changed, new workers will have to be employed and trained, new relationships will have to be developed with other health workers, liaison relationships with other organized nursing services will be necessary, and coordination of community nursing services will be imperative.

Making Referrals and Collaborating with Others in Behalf of the Family

In implementing the nursing care plan, the availability and accessibility of resources and facilities in the community must be kept in mind. The community health nurse has the responsibility to help the family benefit from the services of the available community resources and to interpret and clarify the type and kind of services that are available. Nursing does not have the competencies to meet all the needs of families and must be constantly alert to opportunities for the necessity of referrals to other resources. Making referrals involves a determination of the extent to which nursing can alleviate the need in contrast to the possible contributions of other persons and resources. For example, a family member who has suffered a cerebral vascular accident may need to have rehabilitation services. The nurse may have to make the determination as to whether rehabilitative nursing services will meet his needs, whether a physical therapist is necessary, or whether he should be referred to a rehabilitation center. Her decisions will depend in part upon the community services that are available, but she must weigh all the alternatives as she implements the nursing care plan. If the patient receives only rehabilitative nursing care, will he be able to reach his full potential for rehabilitation? Rehabilitative nursing may help the patient resume the activities of daily living and permit him to stay at home, but is this the ultimate goal for the patient? If it is not, then the nurse will be doing a disservice to the patient and family by not referring him to a physical therapist or to a rehabilitation center.

The amount and kind of nursing service that is needed must also be evaluated. For example, if rehabilitative nursing services can help the patient meet his full rehabilitation potential, how many visits are necessary, how often, and who can best provide them? If daily visits are required but only two visits per week can be made, what will be the final result? If the family and its needs are the focus for service, rather than the needs of the nurse or of the agency, these questions might be more amenable to a solution.

What happens to a family because of visits by a community health nurse? The nurses themselves can give examples of the value of nursing visits, but there has been no concerted, organized effort to document what value has accrued to families because of the nursing input. At the present time there is much discussion but minimal action centered around the need for documented evidence of what happens to families as a result of service by a community health nurse. These discussions have accelerated as a result of some of the definitions of the levels of nursing care which have been developed by third-party payers. Many are geared primarily to the person with an acute illness and do not take into consideration the skilled nursing care needed for the surveillance and maintenance of the health status of individuals and families, or of the anticipatory guidance which is the armamentarium of the community health nurse. Unquestionably, many of the nursing needs of families visited by the community health nurse do not require skilled nursing care, and their require-ments could be met with some kind of custodial nursing care. At the same time there are many families in the community who need skilled nursing care but are not receiving it. It is imperative for community health nursing to differentiate between the need for skilled and custodial nursing care and to develop some immediate and long-range goals to meet these two kinds of nursing needs of people in the community. The plan must also include how to reach the persons who have nursing needs, but who are not receiving nursing service.

The entire nursing process, and particularly the implementation and evaluation steps, are positive action toward analyzing critically the contribution nursing can make to families and the outcomes of various nursing actions. The attitude of community health nurses has been that every family has some health need and undoubtedly could profit from nursing visits. This attitude, however, is no longer tenable in this era of scarcity of health manpower. Increasingly, community health nurses are going to be accountable for the value of their services and must bear full responsibility for demonstrating why their service to families is necessary.

Coordinating the Nursing and Health Services to the Family

The rapid rate at which new knowledge is emerging and the increasing development of technology are the major reasons for the need for specialists in all areas of endeavor today. Thus, we are seeing many persons who are highly skilled and knowledgeable in only one small aspect of a field, with little or no understanding of the field as a whole or of any of the other fields in which persons are involved. The health field, in which new specialists are appearing almost overnight, is a good example of the increasing specialization. Nursing, which has long been influenced by medicine, is also developing highly knowledgeable and skilled specialists. In addition to the increased specialization in the health field, each of the specialists has discovered the community and the family as his arena for practice. As a result, many specialists and specialized health services are available to the people. However, because of the uninhibited proliferation of personnel and services, there are many gaps, with little or no services available in some areas, and in others much overlapping, duplication, and wasted effort.

The community health nurse, with her education and professional commitment geared to the family as the patient, rather than to one age or disease category, can be called a "generalized specialist." She is in a key position to assume the role as primary care nurse to the family, to refer it to other specialists or specialized services as needed, and to coordinate all the health services for the benefit of the family as a whole. For example, when the needs of the family indicate that a specialist in psychiatric nursing or pediatric nursing is necessary for the alleviation of a specific problem, she refers the family member to the nursing specialist in that area. Or if the services of a social worker, nutritionist, physical therapist, and others are necessary, she refers the family member to these persons and resources. She then coordinates the services of the specialists and specialized services with all the other health services the family members are receiving as they relate to the total family situation.

In the early part of the century many nurses were employed by a variety of health organizations, and provided a specialized service to people in their own homes. Thus, we saw tuberculosis nurses, baby nurses, and communicable disease nurses, to name a few. Each had a special interst in one segment of the family and concentrated her efforts in that direction. Usually there was no communication between the nurses or coordination of the nursing services rendered, and the advice given to the family by one nurse often conflicted with that of another. By the twenties many of the public health nursing services to families were of this specialized nature. The effect of this kind of service on families proved to be chaotic, and it was imperative that changes be made. It was at this time that the concept of the family as a unit of service for public health nurses was conceived. As this concept developed, public health nursing services became increasingly generalized, with one nurse providing all the nursing services to the family. The specialized nurses in turn became consultants to the generalized nurse and helped her to utilize their specialized knowledge and skill as she worked with families.

Today we seem to be going through a phase similar to the early part of the century, with many nursing specialists providing services to families. Often these services are provided with little or no coordination with other services the family is receiving. In this context, for example, a mother who has had triplets—one of which may be mentally retarded, one which may have cystic fibrosis, and the other who may be normal—could conceivably have three different nurses visiting her because of three different conditions. No studies have been reported about the effect of specialized, uncoordinated nursing services on families, but we all know of situations in which families have been disrupted and confused as a result. Other questions are being asked about what happens to a family when it must relate to many different professional workers.

The need for coordination of nursing services to families today is analogous to that of the early twenties. At that time, however, as the family became the unit of service for the public health nurse, it was possible to think of one public health nurse with the help of specialized consultants providing all the nursing services needed by a family. In today's society it is impossible for any one individual to have all the knowledge and skill to meet the needs of families. Thus, community health nurses as well as other nursing specialists are being forced to define their particular area of competence. Nursing can no longer be "all things to all people." The focus must be on the health problems and nursing needs of the individual and the family and how these needs can best be met. The community health nurse, with her competence in the area of the family as a whole, must share meaningful information about the family with other disciplines and other nursing specialists; she must refer the families to whatever source can meet their needs; and she must coordinate her services with the other services the family is receiving.

Participating in Continuing Professional Development

The community health nurse has responsibility for her own continuing professional development. In this era of rapid change in all areas of society, knowledge and skill can become obsolete in a very short time. DeCarlo,[1] in discussing the effects of technology on our lives, has said that in a technologic society the emphasis is on knowledge, and that the future belongs to those who study for it and continue an attitude of life-long learning. The necessity for keeping up with new knowledge and practices has been recognized by all health workers as well as by nursing. There is much discussion and some movement toward requiring satisfactory participation in continuing education programs as a prerequisite for renewal of licensure for professional practice. Universities have established and expanded continuing education programs, Regional Medical Programs are intimately involved in continuing education for a wide variety of health workers, and full use is being made of technologic developments. Closed-circuit television, telephone conferences, films, videotapes, and programmed instruction are utilized to provide educational opportunities for health workers to improve their professional practices and to keep abreast of new knowledge in their field.

In addition to pursuing continuing education programs, the community health nurse can keep abreast of new developments in nursing and in the community by such activities as membership in professional organizations, attendance at professional meetings, participating in institutes or workshops, reading the professional literature, and involvement with other health professionals in case conferences, team meetings, and in-service programs.

Nothing can replace the knowledge and skill of the community health nurse in implementing the nursing care plan. How her responsibilities will be carried out and the emphasis given to each responsibility will depend primarily upon the needs of the family, the setting in which the nurse is employed, and the availability of other health team members. Irrespective of these considerations, the process will remain essentially the same.

---

[1] DeCarlo, C. R. Perspectives on Technology. In Ginsberg, E., ed., *Technology and Social Change*. New York, Columbia University Press, 1964, Ch. 1, p. 29.

Evaluation of the Nursing
Care Plan

In today's complex, dynamic society with the increasing demands from the people for more relevent health services, the need for evaluation takes on even greater significance than ever before. The contribution, or lack of contribution, of professional workers is being scrutinized very critically by the people, and searching questions are being asked about why the contributions of professional groups are not meeting the societal needs. At the same time, as even greater strides are made in scientific and technologic developments, there is a concomitant rise in the expectations of the people, with new needs and greater demands being made even before the former ones have been met.

In this pulsating, changing scene, the utilization of available and potential health manpower to meet the present and emerging needs looms as a high-priority item. New professional responsibilities and expanding roles are emerging, and new workers are appearing almost daily. The competencies of each health worker are the hub from which his contributions emanate. Thus, an evaluation of the contributions each worker makes to the solution of health problems of individuals and groups is one of the keys to effective utilization of health manpower. Recent federal health legislation, with built-in requirements for measuring program effectiveness, has given added impetus to the necessity for evaluation of programs and the contribution of health workers.

Evaluation, although listed as the final step in the nursing process, is built in all along the way as the component parts of each step are looked at separately. When short- and long-range goals are stated in relation to behaviors that can be observed and measured, the criteria for evaluation are inherent and clearly evident. By using the evaluative criteria as road signs toward reaching the nursing goals, new vistas of professional responsibility and accountability are opened up, and evaluation becomes an exciting part of the nursing process. The family and its health problems become the focal point for evaluation, rather than the nurse and what she does or does not do. Unquestionably, changes in the health behavior of families are greatly influenced by the imagination, skill, judgment, and knowledge of the nurse; thus, the observed behavior of the family is one indication of the effectiveness of the nurse in working with families.

Some of the time-honored criteria for evaluation, such as how the nurse writes her records, how she organizes her work, her personal appearance, whether she follows agency policies, or whether she accepts criticism well, do not give any indication of what happens to families because of her services. These criteria, however, may have some bearing on how she works with families and how they respond to her.

In addition to the inherent, ongoing, continuous built-in evaluative mechanisms in each step, it is also important to evaluate the total nursing care plan in relation to the health problems and nursing needs of families. Evaluation of the total plan makes it possible to systematically document areas where nursing makes a difference and where it does not make a difference, and to more clearly define problem areas in which nursing research is indicated.

The main concern in evaluating the nursing care plan is whether the nursing goals were reached by the family. If they were reached, one of the questions which must be answered is, "Would the goals have been met without nursing intervention?" This is a vital question and gets at the heart of the cause and effect of nursing intervention. Throughout this book a nursing need has been defined as the contribution nursing can make to the solution of a health problem. This presupposes that in the early steps of the nursing process, family health problems and nursing needs were identified correctly. If, however, the final evaluation indicates that the health problems would have been resolved without nursing intervention, it raises some questions about the accuracy of the identified nursing needs. If it can be documented that the same nursing goals in other families under different situations have been met consistently without nursing intervention, appropriate changes should be made in community health nursing practices.

Another question for which answers must be sought is, "Were the outcomes which accrued from reaching the goals worth the effort, time, and money?" Would a little more or a little less effort or emphasis have made any difference? For example, one of the nursing goals in a family with a mentally retarded child may have been for the child to learn how to feed and dress himself. The nursing action included bi-weekly visits by the nurse. The evaluation could reveal that if daily visits had been made for the first 2 or 3 weeks, the outcomes would have accrued sooner, and at the same time the ability of the family to cope with the problem and to seek help when needed would have been strengthened. As a result, only minimal follow-up visits by the nurse would have been necessary. A critical evaluation of the amount of nursing service expended in relation to the value of the outcomes received will provide some needed guidelines for setting priorities for nursing service.

In reaching the goals, were there any unanticipated outcomes, either positive or negative? It is inevitable that nursing actions in a family will lead to some unanticipated changes in family behaviors. An example of a positive effect is the following: A nursing goal is stated for an obese teen-age daughter to lose 15 to 20 pounds in 6 months. The daughter reaches the goal, and at the same time the diet and eating patterns of the total family improve. An example of an unexpected negative effect could occur from a goal which was geared to keeping an ill member at home. Because of the need of the ill member for a great deal of attention, the needs of the other members are neglected. As a result signs of family disequilibrium appear, such as truancy from school and increased absence from the home. By evaluating why these side effects occur, the role of the nurse as an initiator of behavioral change will be more clearly understood.

If the nursing goals are not reached, the reasons must be ascertained. The reality of the goals for the family should be carefully considered. It may be that the ability of the family to solve its own problems was overestimated and that too much was expected from it at this particular time. As a result the nursing actions were inappropriate and tended to raise the anxiety level of the family. On the other hand, the goals may have been realistic but something happened along the way which changed the family's commitment to them. The clues indicating the changes in commitment were not evident or were not recognized.

The actions of the community health nurse provide the key to whether the nursing goals are met and give evidence of the contribution of nursing to the solution of family health problems. The value of the nursing care plan rests solely upon the resourcefulness and creativity of the nurse as she implements it. What about the nursing actions—were they relevant to the goals and appropriate for the family? The community health nurse must make these distinctions in each family situation. What effect did the timing of the nursing actions have on the attainment of the goals? Oftentimes the idea and the substance of an action is sound, but its effectiveness depends upon the timing, or how and when it was introduced and carried out. Did the nurse have the education and experience to provide the necessary nursing services, to make full utilization of community resources, and to understand the present and future implications of her actions on the family? It may be necessary to increase her competency to work with the family as the patient through participating in in-service education programs, by attendance at workshops and institutes, and by instituting changes in supervisory practices. How did the family feel about the nurse, and how did the members relate to her? The importance of the relationship the community health nurse establishes with the family cannot be underestimated. It is impossible for any one person to relate equally well with everyone. The community health nurse is no exception and must be aware of this and of her effect as a person on the family.

Community health nursing has recognized the necessity for developing criteria to evaluate the quality of nursing services. Nursing administrators are experimenting in various ways with utilization reviews of patient records and with nursing audits. Accreditation of community health nursing programs is another aspect of evaluation. In addition to these administrative endeavors, evaluation must be included as a step in the nursing process and must become an inherent and viable tool for each community health nurse. Only in this way will there be documented evidence of the effectiveness of the contribution of nursing to the solution of family and community health problems.

REFERENCES

American Public Health Association. Glossary of evaluative terms in public health. Amer. J. Public Health, 60:1546-1552, August 1970.

DeCarlo, C. R. Perspectives on Technology. In Ginsberg, E., ed., Technology and Social Change. New York, Columbia University Press, 1964, Ch. 1, pp. 9-43.

Doster, D. D. Utilization of available "nurse power" in public health. Amer. J. Public Health, 60:25-37, January 1970.

George, M., Ide, K., and Vamberg, C. The comprehensive health team: A conceptual model. J. Nurs. Admin., 1:9-13, March-April 1971.

Jones, M. C. An analysis of a family folder. Nurs. Outlook, 16:48-51, December 1968.

National Commission on Community Health Services. Health Is a Community Affair. Cambridge, Mass., Harvard University Press, 1967.

Phaneuf, M. C. Nursing audit for evaluation of patient care. Nurs. Outlook, 14:51-54, June 1966.

Roberts, D., and Hudson, H. How to Study Patient Progress. Public Health Service Publication No. 1169, Washington, D. C. Government Printing Office, 1964.

Ruano, B. J. This I believe . . . about nurses innovating change. Nurs. Outlook, 19:416-418, June 1971.

Schwartz, D. R. Toward more precise evaluation of patient's needs. Nurs. Outlook, 13:42-44, May 1965.

Stewart, R., and Graham, J. Evaluation tools in public health nursing. Nurs. Outlook, 16:50-51, March 1968.

CHAPTER 10

The Community
as the Patient

Community health nursing has a dual responsibility: that of caring for the family and, likewise, the community. Chapter 5 was concerned with the concept of the family as the patient. The focus now shifts to the other equally important patient of the community health nurse—the community.

Public health nursing early recognized the need to work with others in the community and with the community itself for disease prevention and health promotion, and in the 1920s was the standard-bearer for the improvement and expansion of health services. This same broad approach to community health is equally as valid today as it was then—the situation, however, has changed. The concept of the community as the most fruitful arena for improving the health of the people, held for many years primarily by the public health team (nurse, physician, and sanitarian), has now been embraced by an ever-increasing array of health and health-related workers. The community has been given highest priority, and all eyes seem to be turned in its direction. It has become the focal point for interaction for the growing army of concerned and involved health workers and for the myriad of new and expanding health programs.

The time has long since passed when any single profession or group can work alone, chart its own course, and determine its own role. The challenge of finding new and innovative solutions to the complex problems of today's dynamic society offers a real challenge to all health workers. Community health nursing recognizes its share of the burden of responsibility, and is finding new and better ways to contribute its professional knowledge and experience toward the solution of changing health problems. Increasingly, it is taking leadership for nursing in the community, is identifying and interpreting nursing needs to other disciplines, and is collaborating in planning for community health. It recognizes, also, its need to become more knowledgeable about the community itself, and the factors and forces within it—such as power and politics, legislation and financing, leadership and decision making, health issues and action planning, and finally, community change—all of which affect health and health planning. The sphere of action for community health nursing is and must be the broader community itself, rather than the program of any one specific agency.

The word *community* is so frequently used today, in such a variety of contexts, and by people with such different frames of reference, that its meaning has become blurred and nebulous. According to Sanders[1] the community may be viewed in three ways—as a place, as a social system, and as a collection of people. Each has relevance to health.

The view of the community as a place is important for community health nursing. Environment, housing, and transportation are all related to geographic location, as are population composition and distribution, health services, resources, and facilities. Statistical and epidemiologic studies are frequently based on data from specific localities or circumscribed communities. Of increasing importance to all health workers is knowledge of political and legislative jurisdiction, including census tracts and regions—all area-based.

A community can also be viewed as a social system, with its own pattern of interaction which has resulted from the interrelationship of many systems within the community. The community is actually

[1] Sanders, I. T. Public Health in the Community. In Freeman, H. E., Levine, S., and Reeder, L. G., eds., *Handbook of Medical Sociology.* Englewood, New Jersey, Prentice-Hall, Inc., 1965, p. 369.

a combination of all the social units and systems which have been developed to carry out the major functions of the community. Sanders, in describing health as one of the major community systems, states:

> A major community system, whether it be education or the economy, has identifiable characteristics, such as (1) a structure, or a related series of agencies, organizations, or establishments; (2) a set of functions, both manifest and latent; (3) functionaries, or persons charged with the responsibility of promoting the interest of the system or major segments of it; (4) ideology or rationale, which provides the justification for the continuation of the system; (5) paraphernalia, or the necessary equipment and material resources for carrying out the expected activities; and (6) linkages with other systems within and without the community.[2]

Finally, the concept of the community as a collection of people is an extremely important one for health workers.

> The difference between the treatment of disease in an ill individual and planning for improved health for groups of people has been summed up clearly by Carl Taylor. Since the "patient" is a group, pulse and temperature readings are a series of statistical measurements: birth rates, death rates, incidence of particular diseases. Says Dr. Taylor, "Such indices require a basic readjustment in thinking. A woman is either pregnant or not pregnant; a community is about 3 per cent pregnant. A patient has or does not have heart disease; the community always has heart disease, though the rate may go up or down."[3]

A form of community exists wherever a group of people band together for their mutual protection and common good, or to buy and sell their services. The community, therefore, is in reality not buildings, organizations, or a geographic area. It is people—people who are transmitters of value systems and culture, of attitudes toward health and illness, and who vary in a myriad of ways as to ethnicity, social class, education, religion, and health. Klein defines community as:

> patterned interaction within a domain of individuals seeking to achieve security and physical safety, to derive support at times of stress, and to gain selfhood and significance throughout the life cycle. . . . The definition rests on interactions of individuals rather than on social organizations whose nature and functions are a manifestation of those interactions. The term "domain" is used to refer both to a physical place that can be geographically located and to a social-psychological place (such as a community of interest) that

[2] *Ibid.*, p. 375.
[3] Mattison, B. F. Community health planning and the health professions. *Amer. J. Public Health*, 58:1019, June 1968.

> is "phenomenologically real" to those who inhabit it. Community as viewed here, is not man's habitat; rather, it is man-in-habitat, for a habitat is not meaningful without inhabitants.[4]

This fact was graphically illustrated in a recent radio announcement to the effect that it is now possible to purchase, at a relatively low cost, an entire deserted town in a midwestern state—a town complete with houses and schools, streets and transportation, and other community resources. The forces of urbanization were too strong for this town. This is not a community. There are no people. Conversely, strip the inhabitants of a community of all the goods and services available and necessary to them, and they will not survive for very long. John Alexander provides another illustration in his description of Oshkosh, Wisconsin:

> A city is like a living organism. It has a shape and a form—a skeleton, so to speak, of streets, city limits, blocks and buildings. But a city is more than that. A city has life. It has people circulating, in, through, and around those features which constitute its skeleton. Without its people Oshkosh would be dead. To be sure, the streets would still be there; the factories, the stores, the schools, the parks would all be in their same location. Perhaps from the air it would still look like Oshkosh, but it would not be Oshkosh. It is the people who make a city. They constitute the life that ebbs and flows through the inanimate framework.[5]

Klein further emphasizes the importance of community as follows:

> This community, even in today's world of rapid mobility and urban sprawl, is a highly important habitat of man. For it is through community that man is fed and housed, seeks work, educates his children, and in a variety of ways maintains his safety and security. It is also through the community that man discovers problems and their solutions, finds spiritual sustenance, exercises his desire for significant participation in life, and occasionally achieves the highest levels of self-actualization and fulfillment.[6]

There are a variety of approaches which may be used to gather information about a community and contribute to an understanding of its dynamics. Communities, like families, have their own patterned interaction between individuals, families, groups, and organizations, which varies from community to community depending upon the characteristics, needs, and value systems of the population. It is not easy to capture this sense of interaction within a specific community.

[4] Klein, D. C. The meaning of community in a preventive mental health program. *Amer. J. Public Health*, 59:2005, November 1969.
[5] Alexander, J. W. *The Economic Life of Oshkosh.* Madison, University of Wisconsin, Bureau of Community Development, Vol. 5, No. 1 and 2, 1955, pp. 23-24.
[6] Klein, D. C., *op. cit.,* p. 2005.

One way to explore a community is to look at some of the generally accepted functions which it provides for its people. These are:

1. Housing, shelter, use of space
2. Employment, means of livelihood
3. Safety, security, protection
4. Distribution of goods and services
5. Education for children and newcomers
6. Provision of opportunities for interaction between individuals and groups
7. Transmitting information, ideas, beliefs
8. Creating and enforcing rules or standards of beliefs and behavior

A study of any one of these functions results in a great deal of knowledge, much of which is pertinent to health. For example, investigation of the whole problem of housing in low-income, industrial communities results in information about types, conditions, and adequacy of housing, as well as crowding, sanitation, safety, and health. Through further study one is able to collect data concerning public health laws relating to housing and urban development, as well as information about plans for the future.

Another way to learn more about a community is to study its formal organizations or systems. For example, a study of its health organization enables one to determine the number and kinds of its health resources and programs, and the formal interconnecting channels of interagency relationships and communication which have been established. However, systematic study of a community's functions or systems does not necessarily result in greater understanding of community dynamics.

Study of informal as well as formal organization is extremely important and should not be neglected. It is often through knowledge of informal community interrelationships that one learns about how people react, communicate, and solve their problems. Without this understanding one can never hope to develop meaningful, realistic health programs. Community health nursing, in attempting to better understand these dynamics must try to find answers to such questions as:

1. How are decisions made in a particular community? Who makes or who vetoes them? Is there a group of decision makers, or do one or two individuals have the final authority?
2. Where do people go when they are sick or in trouble? Do they use appropriate or inappropriate community resources? Do they go to the doctor, the druggist, or rely on their neighbors?

3. What are the value systems within a community? Where do health and education stand in relation to other community concerns? What has priority?

4. How does the community view change? How have changes come about in the past? What implications does this have for the present and the future?

Our main concern as professional nurses is health. Health, however, has high priority in one community and may be at the bottom of the list in another. Food has the highest priority for the hungry. The fact that communities differ makes it all the more imperative for us to know more about how individual communities view health and change, and why they fail to utilize more effectively many of the services and personnel now available to them. How the people try to meet their health needs, where they go when they are in trouble, and whether they reject or accept help are things that community health nursing must know in order to work effectively.

However we in community health nursing view the community, we must become increasingly knowledgeable about its functions, uniqueness, dynamics, values, characteristics, needs, and most important, about the process by which we can work most effectively with it as our patient. The community is the people, and people are our concern. The community is where planning, with resultant decisions of greatest importance to health, is carried out. The community is where the action is in relation to new, innovative, evolving, and changing health programs and services. It is where community health problems are identified and where significant programs of health promotion and disease prevention, as well as control of major health problems, must be carried out. The community, itself in the process of change, is also the most effective place in which it is possible to bring about change for positive health.

John Gardner, in discussing the Great Society, reminds us that, "Every great creative performance since the initial one has been in some measure a bringing of order out of chaos."[7] To bring order out of chaos is a major task of all who are concerned with health. Americans have the knowledge and the resources, but have not been able or willing to implement a flexible, economically feasible plan of health organization through which quality service can be made available to all who need it. Our heritage of democracy and individualism, coupled with the complexity of an urban society, makes the task of planning quality care a herculean one. Whether this can be done depends more on our wisdom and intelligence than on money or words.

[7]Gardner, J. Gardner hews out the Great Society. *Newsweek*, February 28, 1966, p. 30.

Community health nursing has an important contribution to make to the development of a better health care system. The responsibility for identifying community nursing needs with others, and planning ways in which these needs can be met, rests squarely with community health nursing. This makes obvious the fact that nursing must become increasingly knowledgeable about, and intimately involved in, the planning and decision-making process—of such high priority in today's world.

Often, before community planning can be carried out answers must be found in preplanning to such questions as: Who is the most appropriate person, group, or agency to take leadership within a community, and under what sanction? How is a community problem or need identified and singled out of the complex of possibilities? What has priority? What factors need to be considered—power groups, politics, vested interests—in delineating a plan? What are the resources of the broader region, as well as the individual community? How will the plan be financed? What are realistic long- and short-term goals? What chances of success has a particular plan?

There was little direct governmental encouragement for the process of planning until the 89th Congress passed two laws: Public Law 89-293, Regional Medical Programs, commonly referred to as the heart, cancer, and stroke law; and Public Law 89-749, the Comprehensive Health Planning Act. By enacting these laws the federal government gave direct support to the concepts of preplanning and comprehensiveness. Hilleboe,[8] in editorializing about the administrative process of comprehensive health planning, portrays the essential elements of this process as four triads which are interdependent, interrelated, and interacting. The first triad, the key one, embraces all the problems of community health. Under this he includes mental and physical ailments, environmental hazards to health, and health-related social problems. The second triad includes the types of resources needed to do something about health problems—such as money, manpower, and material. The third triad, community constraints and initiatives, consists of authorizations, norms, and attitudes that are so influential in community health planning. The fourth triad, the planning process itself, embodies administration, the scientific method, and processed data.

This whole process of comprehensive health planning results in decision making. The decisions made at this overall preplanning or planning level are of the greatest importance to both the community

[8]Hilleboe, H. E. Editorial. Concepts of comprehensive health planning. *Amer. J. Public Health*, 58:1001-1002, June 1968.

and its caretakers. It is not only appropriate but imperative that nursing participate with others in the community at the decision-making level in setting directions for the future.

The most stable characteristic of the present health care system is change, characterized by expansion, experimentation, and confusion! Traditional patterns for the delivery of health care are no longer adequate for the twentieth and twenty-first centuries, although many health professionals have been slow either to realize or to admit this fact. We are in the midst of a health care revolution which has come about as the result of far-reaching and rapid societal changes and developments. To name a few: America as an affluent society can afford high quality health care, and this is the right of all citizens, no longer just a privilege; a socially conscious people has declared war on poverty; increasing urbanization has resulted in an urgent demand for new patterns of health service; rapid technologic and scientific developments and new knowledge have made possible and urgent newer methods of treatment and patterns of care; a better-educated and informed public knows what kind of care is possible and demands this care; more people are participating in decision making and asserting the what, where, how, and who regarding community health services; the lines between specialization and generalization are more sharply drawn, while those between care and cure are becoming blurred; and the federal government, increasingly sensitive to the social welfare needs of the country, has responded directly to the urgent demands of the people for better health care.

It is probably safe to say that never before in the history of our country have so many people been concerned about and involved in the community and its problems, including its health problems. No health worker today needs to be reminded of the proliferation of new, different, comprehensive, specialized, reorganized, or combined health programs. He is probably deeply involved in developing one himself. Model cities programs, comprehensive health centers, community mental health centers, store-front clinics, prepaid insurance group practice plans, to name only a few, are multiplying. Many of these new programs are creative and innovative and have resulted in broader and improved care. They have, however, also resulted in disruptions as well as gaps, overlaps, and duplication of previously existing services—and considerable confusion about who does what. At this point in time no one is quite sure just who is responsible for what. This uncertainty creates both excitement and frustration.

There are no ground rules. There are, however, fewer people watching from the sidelines and more in the arena—the community.

Community health nursing is deeply concerned about the community and its health. It is a charter member of the growing group of professionals, semiprofessionals, and other community health workers. More knowledge is available and must be encompassed by this expanding team. Much has been learned about community from social science studies and research. More is known about the relationship between poverty and health. The fact that without intervention the sick get poorer, and the poor get sicker, is beyond dispute, and it is a certainty that health does not exist apart from the social system. No individual, group, or profession can be expert in assessing the complexity of total community health. Each looks at the community from a different vantage point and with its own unique frame of reference and bias. Community health nursing can make its contribution by: identifying factors related to health maintenance, prevention of disease, and promotion of health; identifying and interpreting nursing needs in their relationship to broader community health needs; and planning with others for their solution. Its specific concern with health may be the point of entry which gives it the opportunity to become involved with others in helping to solve some of the broader social problems of the times.

The goals of public health have changed and broadened over the years in relation to developments in medical science and technology, the social and political progress of the country, and the rising aspirations of the people. Early definitions of public health were concerned primarily with sanitary controls for the protection of the individual against health hazards with which he was unable to cope—such as unsafe food and water, and communicable disease. Winslow's definition of public health, written many years ago, is stated in such broad and flexible terms that it is still useful for today and the future:

> Public Health is the Science and Art of (1) preventing disease, (2) prolonging life, and promoting health and efficiency through organized community effort for
> a. the sanitation of the environment,
> b. the control of communicable infections,
> c. the education of the individual in personal hygiene,
> d. the organization of medical and nursing services for the early diagnosis of preventive treatment of disease, and
> e. the development of the social machinery to insure everyone a standard of living adequate for the maintenance of health, so orga-

nizing these benefits as to enable every citizen to realize his birth-right of health and longevity.[9]

A key phrase in this definition is "through organized community effort." If Winslow, often referred to as the father of public health, were writing this definition today, he would undoubtedly include the concept of comprehensive community health planning, since the age of comprehensive health planning is here and those who are concerned with health must accept it.

The need for programs for the protection of the people against the myriad of physical, emotional, social, and environmental health hazards is just as important today as it ever was. The need for comprehensive health programs for diagnosis, treatment, rehabilitation, disease prevention, and education of the public for health also remains of vital importance. The health programs, however, have changed in relation to priorities of other problems. Poverty, partly the result of urbanization and industrialization, is one of the greatest contemporary problems and can no longer be tolerated in an affluent society. Changes in demography and life expectancy, and advances in medical science are just a few of the factors which have resulted in the high priority given to chronic disease programs and research. Environmental and drug problems are of vital concern. Health, however, is only one aspect of life. It affects and is affected by many other factors. Health needs emerge and change as society changes. They must be identified and accorded appropriate priority within the total health planning framework.

It is inevitable that change will occur within the community—change affecting the whole system of the organization, provision, and delivery of health services, as well as the acceptance and utilization of these services by the people.

Physical changes within any community are constant. Population increase or decrease, and shifts in age distribution and composition are continuous. Transportation changes and developments affect mobility, housing, and utilization of resources. Environmental changes and pollution result in new and pressing health problems and concerns.

Changes within the health system itself, always present, are accelerating with the emergence of new health problems, new knowledge,

---

[9]Winslow, C.-E. A. The untilled field of public health. *Mod. Med.*, 2:183, March 1920. Also in Hanlon, J. J., *Principles of Public Health Administration*, 3rd ed., St. Louis, The C. V. Mosby Company, 1960, p. 23.

and an expanding health team. A major factor is the changing role of the government in financing and influencing both health planning and future directions of health care. The relationship between the health system and other community systems is constantly shifting, as national priorities of war and peace, economics, law and order, and education and health shift and change. The whole concept of national health has changed and broadened with positive health a goal, and a national health plan, still on the horizon, nearer to becoming a reality.

Not the least important is the change which has occurred in the consumer of health care. His aspirations for health are high. His knowledge is greater than ever before. He is tired of poor and expensive care, and fragmented services. He is demanding change, and will have it. Robischon, in discussing community health nursing in a changing climate, states:

> We must change our methods and aim our health teaching at populations, rather than individuals. The community nurse of the future, if she is to be skilled as a change agent in promoting health, will need more knowledge about sociocultural patterns, what purposes they serve, how they persist, and how they change. She will also need better understanding of theories of group dynamics, learning, and motivation.[10]

Community health nursing is changing. It is developing new and innovative approaches in providing health services, is focusing more and more on the needs of the community rather than the agency, and is collaborating increasingly with many other concerned workers in planning for the community's health. In this period of specialization, fragmentation, and change, community health nursing is a sustaining force and has a vital role to play in furthering and fostering the health of the community.

The next four chapters are devoted to exploration of the process by which community health nursing works with the community as the patient.

REFERENCES

Alexander, J. W. The Economic Life of Oshkosh. Madison, University of Wisconsin, Bureau of Community Development, Vol. 5, No. 1 and 2, 1955.

[10] Robischon, P. Community nursing in a changing climate. *Nurs. Outlook*, 19:413, June 1971.

Conant, R. W. The Politics of Community Health. National Commission on Community Health Services, Report of the Community Action Studies Project, Washington, D. C., Public Affairs Press, 1968.

Fifer, E. Z. Hang-ups in health planning. Amer. J. Public Health, 59:765-769, May 1969.

Freeman, H. E., Levine, S., and Reeder, L. G., eds. Handbook of Medical Sociology. Englewood, N. J., Prentice-Hall, Inc., 1963.

Gardner, J. Gardner hews out the Great Society. Newsweek, February, 28, 1966.

Hanlon, J. J., Principles of Public Health Administration, 3rd ed. St. Louis, The C. V. Mosby Company, 1960.

Harnish, T. I. Regional medical program planning. Amer. J. Public Health, 59:770-772, May 1969.

Hilleboe, H. E. Editorial. Concepts of comprehensive health planning. Amer. J. Public Health, 58:1001-1002, June 1968.

——Public health in the United States in the 1970's. Amer. J. Public Health, 58:1588-1610, September 1968.

Klein, D. C. Community Dynamics and Mental Health. New York, John Wiley and Sons, Inc., 1968.

——The meaning of community in a preventive mental health program. Amer. J. Public Health, 59:2005-2012, November 1969.

Lewis, C. E. The thermodynamics of regional planning. Amer. J. Public Health, 59:773-777, May 1969.

Mattison, B. F. Community health planning and the health professions. Amer. J. Public Health, 58:1015-1021, June 1968.

Mott, B. J. The myth of planning without politics. Amer. J. Public Health, 59:797-803, May 1969.

Polk, L. D. Areawide comprehensive health planning: The Philadelphia story. Amer. J. Public Health, 59:760-764, May 1969.

Robischon, P. Community nursing in a changing climate. Nurs. Outlook, 19:410-413, June 1971.

Sanders, I. T. The Community. New York, The Ronald Press Company, 1958.

Sheahan, M. W. Through community action: A health commission reports. Amer. J. Nursing, 66:1298-1302, June 1966.

Smolensky, J., and Haar, F. Principles of Community Health. Philadelphia, W. B. Saunders Company, 1961.

Winslow, C-E.A. The untilled field of public health. Mod. Med., 2:183, March 1920. Also in Hanlon, J. J., Principles of Public Health Administration. St. Louis, The C. V. Mosby Company, 1964.

CHAPTER 11

Gathering Pertinent Data
About the Community

The community health nurse participates with professional and lay persons in identifying the factors within the community relevant to health. She collaborates in planning, implementing, and evaluating the community health program, and assumes leadership in interpreting nursing data and defining nursing needs. The first step in this process involves collection of pertinent information about the community.

Community health nurses have a great deal of knowledge about their communities. They serve the families who are the community, and interact with many individuals, groups, and organizations in their behalf. They know the people, neighborhoods, streets, and resources. They participate on innumerable committees, both as professional nurses and as citizens. They have access to records, studies, annual reports, and statistics. They talk to people about the community, read about it, observe it, spend a good deal of their time in it, and

205

obviously have a storehouse of valuable information. Too often, unfortunately, this wealth of knowledge is neither reported, assembled, nor documented. Too often it is hidden away in different and widely scattered files, with the result that when one tries to assess the needs of a community, information which could be most valuable is not available, and important decisions are often made on the basis of inadequate data.

What kinds of information are important for assessment of community nursing needs? This may appear to be a simple question, but the answer is far from simple. There is no general agreement about the breadth or depth of knowledge that is specific for the determination of health problems of a community, of which nursing needs are an inherent part. However, the authors believe that there are certain kinds of factual information about a community which provide an overall picture and serve as a framework for the identification of the health problems from which nursing needs are determined. These kinds of information include:

1. Data about the community itself—its physical characteristics, uniqueness, and personality.

2. Information about the people—their distribution and characteristics.

3. Knowledge about the environment—the housing, air and water, safety, and health-related factors.

4. Knowledge about the channels of communication, both formal and informal, and the key communicators within the community.

5. Vital statistics and information about the population—its health and illness patterns and problems.

6. Data about the health and health-related facilities, resources, and personnel.

7. Knowledge about available community health nursing services and programs—their resources and interrelationships.

Much of this kind of information is important to many different health workers as well as to community health nursing. Of significance, however, is: how each professional group such as doctors, social workers, community health nurses, and social scientists interprets this information in light of its professional frame of reference and knowledge; what additional questions each asks; and how each utilizes this knowledge as the basis for determination of future action. Herein lies the uniqueness and potential contribution of each professional group.

Community health nursing in studying the community should first find out whether pertinent and related studies have already been done, what kinds of information and health data these provide, and what additional information is available from key people and resources, including community health nursing itself. Any other knowledge deemed necessary to provide a more total picture of the community can then be obtained. These data which have been assembled must be ordered and organized in such a way as to be useful for analysis. Therefore, community health nursing needs to develop a profile of the community being studied, so that the multitude of factors relating to both its health and nursing needs can be viewed in their proper perspective and relationship. The authors have developed a suggested community nursing survey guide[1] to assist in the collection, compilation, and organization of data, and the development of a profile.

Anyone involved in a community study must be sensitive to the desires, needs, and values of each community, and modify his approach appropriately. All this directly affects how data are collected and to what extent. The process of gathering pertinent and basic data about a community and its people, however, remains the same whether the community is a county, a city, a census tract, the area covered by a nursing organization, or the district of an individual community health nurse.

Data About the Community   How can a particular community best be described? What are the unique characteristics that differentiate it from any other community? Is it an inner-city area or neighborhood of a large urban complex? Is it a middle-class suburb with its own form of town government, or a farming community in the South or Midwest? What about its location, climate, and topography—factors which directly influence both the health needs and the patterns of delivery of health services. What are the specific geographic limits of the community? These need to be defined and described as clearly as possible. Parameters may often be delineated by natural boundaries such as rivers and mountains, as well as by roads, streets, or by census tracts. The use of census tracts as boundaries fits in with the political jurisdiction. There is less chance of duplication, gaps, and overlapping of statistics when census tracts are used. Census tracts

[1] Appendix B.

were initially small areas in a community averaging about 4,000 inhabitants but are now much larger. The boundaries are usually established jointly by local committees and the Bureau of the Census to achieve some homogeneity of such population characteristics as economic status and living conditions.

How large is this community and what is the population per square mile? How is this population distributed spatially? Is it characterized by areas of density and areas of sparcity? This kind of information is extremely important when one is considering the location, distribution, and delivery of health services. It gives clues about some of the kinds of health problems which might be present.

Information about the existing form of government is of increasing significance to health workers. The health of the community is the legal responsibility of the governmental agency—the health department. The more that community health nurses know about the governmental structure affecting health, about how and how much tax money is allocated for health, and the steps necessary for submitting new legislation and supporting or opposing pending legislation, the better they will understand and contribute to the solution of health problems. The federal government has become more and more responsive to the health needs of the nation, and the flow of legislation affecting health continues to increase. This makes paramount an understanding of the relationship of local governing groups to those at the state and federal level.

A brief history of the community is invaluable in these days of slum clearance, urban development, city planning, and major highway construction. The problems encountered by a community involved in any one of these major processes are manifold and disruptive, and demand considerable community adjustment and change. It must be kept in mind that no group or community can adjust too far in any direction without upsetting its state of equilibrium. If change comes about too rapidly, communities are faced at every turn with completely new situations for which they are unprepared.

It is the responsibility of community health nursing, together with other key community workers and institutions, to help a community maintain its equilibrium. Therefore, when major community change is anticipated—change which may be catastrophic to one community yet easily assimilated by another—potential problems must be anticipated and plans for orientation to and preparation for change worked out in advance. Thus, knowledge of what has happened to a community in the past, and knowledge of possible plans for the future give perspective to the present and make possible advance planning. The present always lies between the past and the future and must be viewed in this context.

Information About the People

Certain kinds of data about the population of a community, such as age and sex distribution, ethnic and religious composition, education, and socioeconomic status, should be assembled and considered before any serious assessment of health or nursing needs is attempted.

Knowledge about the percentage of people within each age category contributes to the identification of health needs. What is the proportion of preschool children in relation to the total population? What particular kinds of health services do preschoolers need? Are these currently available? What proportion of community nursing services is directed toward this particular group? Pertinent questions such as these should be asked in relation to each age group within the population.

How many people within the community are 65 years of age and over? This knowledge is important when one is planning for an aging population. The fact that the population is aging has a direct affect upon the whole health picture. In any community with a growing percentage of older people, particular consideration must be given to the gamut of services for prevention and care, the resources necessary for hospital or extended home care, and the supply of supporting personnel so often required by the elderly.

Systematic compilation of information about age and sex of the population does not assure answers about specific health problems. It does, however, give important clues as to possible nursing needs and provides a framework of information within which health needs of specific age groups can be studied and looked at in relation to current programs. Many times, studying the age distribution of a population over a period of time brings to light the fact that there has been a population shift. Accompanying changes in priorities of community nursing services should reflect this shift.

The relationship between the health of a community and a variety of its population characteristics—ethnic, socioeconomic, educational, and religious—is well established. Knowledge of these characteristics is equally as important as that of age and sex distribution. It is a well-known fact that health problems are associated with poverty areas, particularly ghettos—concentrations of predominantly black, socioeconomically and educationally deprived people. Poverty, however, is not limited to the blacks but is the condition of many others across the country, such as the American Indian, the Puerto Rican, the migrant, and the so-called poor white. Population characteristics and distribution give valuable clues as to the population needs of particular groups, and contribute another dimension to the overall assessment of a community. Comparison of the data about income, occupation, and rate of unemployment of one community with that of another can be significant in giving clues as to financial, educational, vocational, and nutritional needs, as well as health needs.

Knowledge About the Environment

The American people have finally awakened, and none too soon, to the sad and sorry plight of their environment, and to the havoc wrought by the accelerating technologic development of the last 150 years—technologic development paralleled by increasing pollution of air, water, and land. The frightening spectre of a rapidly diminishing system of life support on earth is before us. Man's future survival may depend upon his understanding and appreciation of the relationship of organisms (man included) to their environment. Community health nurses, as citizens as well as health workers, must be concerned with the environment of the community.

Housing is more than a roof over one's head. It provides the primary environment for children's growth and development, and for family interaction and relationships. It has a great deal to do with the quality of health and of life. The relationship of inadequate and overcrowded habitation to increased health problems—physical, social, and emotional—has been well documented. Information about the adequacy of living and housing conditions of the families in the community, about safety, overcrowding, sanitation, insect and rodent infestation, and general state of repair of the houses is basic in any study of health problems. Many of the causes of the current housing crisis are due to the fact that there has been failure to enact and enforce many of the housing codes, regulations, and zoning laws which already exist. There has also been lack of foresight in planning for future housing. Additional information about existing housing regulations and the mechanisms for their enforcement should be sought.

The majority of people across the country take for granted a safe, clean, adequate water supply and do not become unduly concerned until there is a drought or some kind of disaster which makes starkly evident the fact that water is a necessity of the highest priority. The supply of water and the regulations for its safety vary, depending upon the type of community. In a rural farming area which uses well water, for example, the problems related to a safe water supply are different from those of an urban community with a municipal water supply. Knowledge about fluoridation will give clues about the dental health problems which might be found in a community.

A workable plan for garbage, trash, and sewage disposal is mandatory for maintenance of human and environmental health. However, because of the mass of disposable and nondestructible material resulting from our way of life, such a plan is difficult to develop. As with water, the problems of waste disposal in urban and rural communities have some striking differences. The concern of a rural community may be a smoking, stinking, rat-infested dump or an overflowing cesspool; while that of an urban area may be trash-littered streets, overturned garbage cans, or overflowing toilets. Sanitary regulations and collection schedules exist in almost every section of the country. Information about the rules, regulations, and standards regarding garbage collection and disposal—and, most important, mechanisms for their enforcement—contributes to the definition of health problems.

Never before in our memory have protective services, such as police, fire, and civil defense been so vital. The ongoing responsibilities of maintaining law, order, safety, and protection have been compounded with additional problems associated with racial tensions, student unrest, demonstrations, drug addiction, and violence. In addition to traditional protective services, other resources and programs are often available to a community. They may include such things as: transportation services to hospitals and clinics; emergency ambulance services; respirator services; and even educational programs concerning such things as alcoholism, drug addiction, and safety. This kind of information is particularly helpful to community health nurses in planning to meet nursing needs.

Although transportation patterns and resources vary from community to community, particularly between urban, suburban, and rural areas, there is a direct relationship between the availability of transportation and the utilization and delivery of health services. The elderly, the ill, the mother with several small children, the poor, the poorly motivated—these and many others are less apt to get to medical facilities if transportation is unavailable, inconvenient, time consuming, or expensive. Lack of parking facilities presents similar difficulties for those with automobiles. Knowledge about transportation routes, frequency of service, costs, transfers, and the transportation problems of any particular segment of the population is essential. In addition, information about planned future changes in transportation patterns, routes, or resources has implications for health planning and may affect decisions about the establishment and location of clinics and other health facilities.

Channels of Communication

Communication, a process by which people exchange ideas and interact, is basic to community life. Within every community there are well-defined formal and informal systems of communication. Informal methods are numerous and tend to operate wherever groups of people collect, such as in hospitals, industries, universities, or wherever conversation is free and easy among people—at the gas station, beauty parlor, or chain store; over the bridge table; or at a neighborhood well-child conference. There are key people within every community who, because of their status or community orientation, are more apt to be an integral part of informal communication which transmits information about local affairs. These key people, or high communicators, should be identified. They can be of great help to health workers and should be involved, whenever feasible, in any community health study.

Formal channels of communication through traditional media such as newspapers, television, radio, telephone, and postal systems are equally important to community life. The press, which includes newspapers, special interest publications, magazines, and community papers, continues to be a powerful means of communicating information, ideas, and attitudes. Television, now found in the majority of American homes, is also of significance. Studies and spot checks of television viewers indicate which segment of the population is most likely to be reached at what time of day and on what days. Such information is valuable to community workers regarding spot announcements in support of local projects or for dissemination of health information. Knowledge about these existing formal and informal channels of communication is essential for better understanding ways in which ideas, attitudes, and knowledge about health are disseminated, and also how they may be used most effectively for health education.

Health and Illness Patterns
The statistics of a community provide data about the vital events that occur in the population, such as births, deaths, and occurrence of disease. The necessity for a systematic collection of vital statistics was recognized by the federal government at the beginning of the century with the establishment of the Death Registration Area in 1900 and the Census Bureau in 1902. Data about the vital events in a population are basic to the development and evaluation of any community health program. They are also indispensable in any study of community health problems. The number and rate of live births that occur only provide information about the number of persons who are born during any specific period of time. However, this information is necessary for effective planning of facilities of all kinds, such as hospitals, nursery schools, schools, housing, recreation facilities, and health facilities. The number of deaths and the death rate give a picture of the number of people who have died and the incidence of various causes of death over a specific period of time. Caution should be used in defining health problems in a community on the basis of the number of deaths, however, and these data should be looked at in relation to many other factors.

A comparison of birth and death rates of one community with those of adjoining communities, the state, or the nation as a whole gives valuable clues about some of the health problems in a particular community and clues as to the effectiveness of the existing health programs. For example, if the maternal death rate in one community is higher than that of surrounding communities and the state as a whole, this alerts the community to the fact that a problem exists and warrants further exploration.

Health Facilities and Resources Health facilities and resources dot our communities like raisins in a fruit cake, but there is real question at this point in time as to whether there is an actual health care system in America. A system suggests some overall plan or organization. The existence of two systems, one for the "haves" and one for the "have nots" is probably nearer the truth.

Until recently, marked separation prevailed generally between curative and preventive services, with little reaching out on the part of the hospitals into the community and, likewise, little coordination of preventive and health promotional services with those of the hospital. Fortunately, dissatisfaction on the part of many—rich and poor, the black and the white, consumer and worker, young and old—about both the availability, quality, and fragmentation of health care is resulting in a movement toward more comprehensive health planning. The rate and manner of planning are about as varied as the communities which exist, and no two of these are alike. Rapid changes have resulted in much confusion, proliferation, overlapping, and duplication of services and will, no doubt, continue for some time to come. It would take more than a skilled clairvoyant to predict the kind of a system that will eventually emerge. There is a consensus, however, about the fact that there will be change to a new pattern of organization of health services. Currently, several models for a possible national health plan are being discussed and considered.

In order to get as clear a picture as possible about a community's health facilities and resources, there must be compilation of information about them and their interrelationships. Data must be gathered about the hospitals, clinics, nursing homes, schools, occupational health programs, comprehensive and neighborhood health centers, model cities programs, prepaid group insurance plans, and other resources significant to health. Kinds of data should include: purposes of programs, types of services, numbers of beds, kinds and numbers of personnel employed, utilization of personnel, and the interrelationships which have developed between and among these various facilities. What about health-related planning groups within the community—such as health or neighborhood councils, councils of health and social agencies, and concerned citizens' groups? Such groups play a vital role in initiating, supporting, and furthering community health. In the last analysis, it is human resources which make all this a reality. In most communities there are human resources in addition to those persons employed in its health agencies. Often nurses, teachers, educators, doctors, social workers, and sociologists—some active and some retired—live within a community and are intimately concerned with its welfare. Faculty from local or neighboring colleges and universities and consultants from state, federal, and other agencies are all important members of a community's human health resources.

Information About Existing Community Nursing Services

If the community health nursing services in many communities could be pictorially portrayed, they would probably look like an old-fashioned crazy quilt, or a collage made up of light and dark oddly shaped patches. Therefore, data about the kinds and extent of available community health nursing services must be collected before any analysis of their adequacy in relationship to need can be attempted. This process includes systematic collection of data about existing community health nursing services. The agency may be voluntary or official, a comprehensive or neighborhood health center, a school, or an occupational health or model cities program. The purpose of each agency studied needs to be clearly stated. For example, while a voluntary nursing program exists for the provision of community nursing services and education, an official agency such as a health department has much broader purposes, with nursing as only one aspect. On the other hand, a neighborhood health center is generally a comprehensive facility providing or arranging for continuous family-centered, preventive, and curative services under one roof for those members of a defined community.

An official agency derives its legal authority from the power of the state through public health law, while a voluntary agency gets its authority by virtue of state incorporation. Authority for the health of school children, however, varies across the country—resting with either the board of health, the board of education, or under joint administration.

In order for an agency to qualify as a certified home health agency under Medicare, certain standards for quality control must be maintained, and the inclusion of at least one secondary service such as physical therapy, occupational therapy, or medical social work is mandatory. Agency certification is of real significance regarding agency program and direction, and community health nursing should be knowledgeable about this.

In 1966 a joint program of accreditation of community nursing services was established by the National League for Nursing and the American Public Health Association. This was the first time that there had been accreditation of any kind for nursing services. This process of accreditation, which includes self-involvement and self-evaluation on the part of the agency, has stimulated and motivated agencies to improve services. It also has given added protection to society for better quality of care. Knowledge of agency accreditation gives one clues as to the quality of service and agency aspirations.

A table of organization of a community health agency provides the basis for a clearer understanding of the relationship of community health nursing to the agency's total program—particularly in regard to authority, responsibility, and channels of communication.

Administrative patterns within organizations are far from uniform, either on the state or local levels, and therefore must be looked at individually. In general, administrative responsibility in voluntary agencies rests with a lay board of directors which has the responsibility for the appointment of an executive director of nurses. On the other hand, administration of a local official agency generally rests with an appointed or locally elected board of health which in turn appoints the health officer. The employment of all other personnel, including nursing, is customarily the prerogative of the health officer (and his advisory committee) but subject to civil service regulations if these exist. Consumer groups are assuming increasing administrative responsibilities for many of the programs in some of the newer kinds of organizations, such as model cities and neighborhood health centers. As previously discussed, administration of school health services varies from health department to department of education to joint administration. Whichever plan prevails, it has a direct effect upon the scope and responsibility of the school health service.

Knowledge of the administrative patterns of an agency such as the composition of its board and advisory committees, its qualifications and standards for appointment of personnel, its channels of communication and processes for decision making, as well as the relationship of nursing within the structure contributes to an understanding of the existing nursing services available to the community.

A job description of the nursing director, including such things as educational qualifications and previous experience, gives important clues as to the value placed on professional nursing by the board and community. It also clarifies the relationship of the nursing administrator to the health officer, the board of directors, consumer groups, or other administrative bodies, and her lines of communication within the agency and community.

Every organization responsible for using either private or public sources of income must be accountable for its funds and should have a realistic, up-to-date budget and a sound system of accounting. According to Hanlon:

> A sound system of accounting serves many purposes. It provides a financial record of the activities of an agency, reveals its financial condition at all times, provides very necessary data upon which the departmental administrator may base plans for future action, gives substantive protection in case of questions, and provides the fundamental starting point for audits.[2]

Budget problems of home health agencies are becoming increasingly complex with the advent of such programs as Medicare, Medicaid, Maternal and Infant Care, Children and Youth, and the expansion of third-party payments and contractual agreements. A great deal can be learned about programs, staffing, services, and priorities within the community by studying the budgets of its community health agencies. Financing of health services gives clues about the value which a community places on health and its willingness to support it financially.

Public health nurses were the first professional group to study the cost of a nursing visit. They have developed a variety of cost study methods. It is helpful to know when an agency's latest cost analysis was done, what method was used, and the charge to the recipient of the service.

The success of any community health nursing program depends upon its personnel—their adequacy, quality, and utilization. Twenty years ago one could quote generally accepted minimal staffing requirements per unit of population for basic health services. This is no longer possible. Patterns for the provision of basic services have changed considerably over the past few years. Nonprofessional and

[2]Hanlon, J. *Principles of Public Health Administration,* 3rd ed. St. Louis, The C. V. Mosby Company, p. 299.

paraprofessional workers, with varying kinds of preparation, have joined the community health team. Clinical specialists are becoming more and more involved in the community. Many hospital-based home care programs have become more comprehensive and have extended their services into the community. Finally, the consumer has broadened his health aspirations and is playing a much more vital role in the whole area of community health. The establishment of a ratio of community health nurses per unit of population is no longer possible or feasible.

The task of gathering information about health manpower resources—and of particular interest to us, community health nursing and its supporting resources—is increasingly difficult. Information about the staffs of community health nursing agencies, as to their qualification and numbers, and about other nursing resources available within the community need to be assembled before any analysis of the situation can even be attempted.

Although knowledge about numbers, kinds, and qualifications of personnel is important, it is of no value unless one looks at the ways in which available personnel are utilized to meet the needs of the community. Study of patterns of utilization gives clues to: priorities of service and rationale for nursing assignments; evidence of application of new knowledge and trends which have developed; kinds of coordination which exist with other community services; and finally, ways in which contributions of an expanding community health nursing team are integrated and utilized.

Data needs to be collected about the services that are offered by the agencies. Who provides bedside care in the community? What about preventive services and health guidance? Are services available for all age groups and disease categories? What percentage of people in a community avail themselves of these services? What kinds of clinics are available, and how are they utilized? How broad are the offerings of the school health program? How is school health coordinated with other nursing programs within the community? What kinds of programs such as community health centers, neighborhood clinics, model cities programs, or prepaid group insurance programs have developed within the community? What nursing services do they offer, and how do these programs relate to other community nursing services? What about any other community programs in which the nurse is involved?

Finally, what patterns and mechanisms for coordination of community health nursing services and what collaborative arrangements, both formal and informal, have been developed within the community? This information can later be studied, as one might study a sociogram, as part of the analysis of community nursing needs. It is through these kinds of arrangements and community relationships that one attempts to tie the resources together into a fabric of community health nursing services which contributes to continuous comprehensive care—the ultimate goal.

This chapter has been concerned with the kinds of data about a community and its people which must be collected and understood by community health nursing as the basis for the next step in the process—analysis of data and identification of nursing needs.

REFERENCES

American Public Health Association. A Self-Study Guide for Community Health Action-Planning, Vols. I and II. New York, American Public Health Association, 1967.

Carnegie Commission on Higher Education. Higher Education and the Nation's Health. New York, McGraw-Hill Book Company, 1970.

Fonaroff, A. Identifying and developing health services in a new town. Amer. J. Public Health, 60:821-828, May 1970.

Fox, J., Hall, C., and Elerback, L. Epidemiology: Man and Disease. New York, The Macmillan Company, 1970.

Hanlon, J. J. Principles of Public Health Administration, 3rd ed. St. Louis, The C. V. Mosby Company, 1960.

Hilleboe, H. E. Public health in the United States in the 1970's, Amer. J. Public Health, 58:1588-1610, September 1968.

McNeil, H. How to become involved in community planning. Nurs. Outlook, 17:44-47, February 1969.

Means, R. Interpreting statistics: An art. Nurs. Outlook, 13:34-37, May 1965.

National Commission on Community Health Services. Health Is A Community Affair. Cambridge, Mass., Harvard University Press, 1967.

Sanders, I. T. The Community. New York, The Ronald Press Company, 1958.

Stewart, D., and Vincent, P. Public Health Nursing. Dubuque, Iowa, William C. Brown Company, Publishers, 1968.

CHAPTER 12

Analysis of Data and Identification of Community Nursing Needs

A community is people. Facts and information about these people, their way of life and health can be assembled, studied, and analyzed. This process of data analysis involves:

1. Analyzing the data for relationships and clues to the community's health status and concerns.
2. Determining the health problems.
3. Identifying the nursing needs.

It would be presumptuous to claim that in order to understand a community one must have all the facts about it. Obviously, this is not possible. One does need, however, to collect data which is broad, significant, and pertinent to the problem at hand—in this instance, community health nursing.

Health is caught in a web of environmental, social, and economic influences. The pathology of poverty, as well as inadequate income, unemployment, disability, and excessive mobility necessitate knowledge of social patterns as well as health data. Because of these interrelationships which affect and are affected by health, community health nursing must have access to broad and basic data about the community, its people, and their health before any meaningful analysis is possible. The National Commission on Community Services[1] has recommended criteria which can be used as a yardstick for the overall health services of a community, including its community health nursing services. They provide a frame of reference within which to look at health services, and should be kept in mind during the analysis. These are:

1. *Health services should be comprehensive.* To be comprehensive, as the term implies, they should provide health care for all the people in the community who need it wherever they need it—in hospitals, clinics, outpatient departments, extended care facilities, in school, in place of work, or in the home.

2. *Health care should be continuous and coordinated.* Health care is defined as encompassing total care of the sick, health guidance, disease prevention and rehabilitation, and care for all age groups. This care may be provided by a great variety of people and institutions, such as private physicians, traditional health care institutions, and official and voluntary community health agencies, as well as by comprehensive and neighborhood health centers, model cities programs, and a myriad of other ways. Irrespective of who provides this care, it should be available to all the people in the community. It should be focused on the needs of the individual, the family, and the community and be continuous and coordinated.

3. *Health care must be available, accessible, and acceptable.* Care may be available to a community as a whole and valuable to those who can or do avail themselves of it. It is of no value, however, for those to whom it is inaccessible or unacceptable, for a complex variety of limitations or reasons.

4. *Health care requires adequate facilities, personnel, and finances.* No community can provide comprehensive care unless it has an adequate amount of all these resources. Communities need to take a long hard look at the places and people who are providing the services and at other, often new and innovative ways in which services can be obtained or provided.

These criteria provide desirable yardsticks against which a community and its health services can be studied. It must always be kept in mind, however, that the data which have been collected about a

[1] National Commission on Community Health Services. *Health Is A Community Affair.* Cambridge, Massachusetts, Harvard University Press, 1967.

particular community must be analyzed in the light of this community's unique characteristics and individual health problems and needs. Since the problems of no two communities are alike, solutions must be individually tailored. This principle is equally applicable in relation to community health nursing, and the nursing needs cannot be determined independently or out of context.

The Community

Descriptive information about the community being studied is invaluable. It immediately gives one "the feel" of the community and a frame of reference within which to proceed. For example, just knowing that the community of concern is an urban ghetto may, it is true, conjure up a stereotype. However, it also gives one valid and realistic clues that a possible pathologic, health-related complex may exist. On the other hand, if the community is an upper-middle-class suburb, a whole different set of possibilities presents itself. The community may be vastly different from either of these. It may be a metropolitan census tract or a sleepy New England village. Descriptive and identifying information about the characteristics of the community, its size, location, topography, climate, and population, provides a frame of reference within which community health nursing can study data and their relationships.

The location of a community has a great deal to do with health. Two very different communities, one an Appalachian settlement isolated by mountains, poor roads, poverty, and cultural privation; and the other, an affluent middle-class suburb firmly connected to a neighboring city by bands of superhighways, will differ in many ways, such as: relationships with neighboring communities; health and health-related problems; availability, accessibility, and utilization of resources; patterns of transportation; socioeconomic and educational levels; and occupational opportunities. Knowledge of geographic location also tells one something about climate and immediately suggests differences in general as well as seasonal patterns of living—such as that of the Deep South in comparison with the Northwest or the New England area.

The relationship between the size or area of a community and its population, particularly the location of its population, is most significant. Clusterings of poor families within certain census tracts or neighborhoods, for example, predict constellations of problems and indicate need for closer scrutiny of health data, facilities, and resource utilization as well as educational levels and opportunities.

Analysis of the mobility patterns of the population is basic to planners of health services. Mobility and length of residence are particularly significant when looked at in relation to other factors, such as socioeconomic, ethnic, occupational, and educational considerations. Data of this kind give one better understanding about the dynamics of a community and clues about possible kinds of approaches which might be most effectively used in health planning and intervention.

Community health nursing is well aware of the changing and increasingly active role and influence of the federal government in relation to both social and health planning and financing. Over the past few years Congress has enacted health legislation with which most health workers are familiar. Some of these are: Comprehensive Health Planning, P.L. 89-749; Regional Medical Programs, P.L. 89-239; the Economic Opportunity Act, P.L. 90-222; and the Demonstration Cities and Metropolitan Development Act, P.L. 89-754, known as the Model Cities Program.

Although a large number of federal agencies conduct and finance health activities, the great proportion is still provided by private, voluntary, independent, and often specialized agencies. The boundary however, between public and private programs is often hazy, and not clearly understood. Therefore, analysis of data about existing governmentally sponsored or funded programs, such as Medicare and Medicaid, helps to clarify parameters, relationships, gaps, duplication, and fragmentation of services.

Many times official programs are planned without adequate involvement of either consumers or other significant and appropriate health workers, including community health nursing. Often, today, there is antagonism against bureaucracy and a desire for community control in the face of inadequate facilities and resources.

Analysis of data about current legislation in a community and about patterns and forms of local government gives knowledge and clues about channels and mechanisms which can be used by those who wish to speak for and against pending legislation and participate in initiating new and additional legislation.

The concept that the past is significant to both the present and the future, a major theme of this book, is directly applicable to analysis of data about a community. Each community, like every individual, adjusts to change in its own unique way. Understanding how change and crisis has been handled in the past makes future behavior more predictable. One community may still be in a state of shock after having recently been bisected by a superhighway. Another community may be struggling with depression and unemployment resulting from a prolonged strike affecting its key industry. An extensive redevelopment program may cause disequilibrium in one community, while another will seemingly "take it in its stride." Analysis of what has happened to a community in the past, when it happened, and how the community was able to cope with change, gives important clues as to its adjustability and dynamics, and possible timing for introduction of further change.

Equally as important as analysis of the history of a community is knowledge of future change. This is of real significance in relation to the assessment of community's strengths and weaknesses and to the timing of anticipated health planning.

Through the foregoing analysis of the information about the community—description, location, population, government and legislative process, history, and future plans—some of the relationships between items in this category have been discussed, and clues as to their meaning and significance to community health nursing suggested. Analysis of data about each and every community will no doubt bring to light the need for further and different questions to be asked and additional facts to be gathered. All this will result in new relationships and broader understanding of the range of ways through which the people may be helped to deal more effectively with their problems.

Population Characteristics

It is evident that analysis of the characteristics of a community's population, the very people in aggregate who give it life and meaning, is of the greatest significance to community health nursing and basic to determination of health problems and nursing needs. The following population characteristics should be explored: age, sex, and race distribution; ethnic group composition; religion; educational levels; and socioeconomic factors.

Population takes on meaning to health workers primarily when it is analyzed in terms of its distribution or component parts. For example, the fact that one section of an urban community being studied has a population of 77,000 is important. Further knowledge that the population has decreased by 11.6 percent over the last 6-year period adds another dimension and suggests that those who could afford to, have moved to better neighborhoods. A look at some of the socioeconomic, occupational, and ethnic characteristics of the community will help to clarify this population shift.

Many clues about possible health needs can be gleaned from studying the age distribution of a population. For example, the age distribution of the population of 77,000, previously referred to, is as follows:

Age Group	Percent of Population
0-19	36.8
20-34	19.0
35-59	28.0
60-64	4.4
65-69	4.1
70-74	3.4
75+	4.3

Possibilities for analysis of this data are manifold. In addition to looking at the overall age distribution and its meaning, one can also focus on each individual segment of the population and study it more definitively. To illustrate, a further breakdown of the age distribution of the younger segment of this population points out that of the 0-19 age group, 32.7 percent is 0-5 years of age; 26.6 percent is 5-9 years of age; 22.4 percent is 10-14 years of age; and 18.3 percent is 15-19. This additional information about the population will need to be studied carefully in relation to vital statistics, health data, and needs pertinent to each age group. It should then be looked at in relationship to socioeconomic, environmental, and cultural factors if it is to have real meaning and relevance to health workers.

Comparison of age distribution of one population with that of a neighboring community, the state, or the country as a whole further pinpoints population differences and predictable concerns. Also, a look at shifts in age distributions in relation to services and resources for each age category may be both revealing and disconcerting.

Knowledge of ethnicity, race, and religion of a population becomes particularly meaningful when any ethnic or religious group is concentrated within a community or in a particular neighborhood. The cultural values, mores, and customs, for example, prevalent in a predominantly Chinese, Irish, Puerto Rican, or Jewish neighborhood directly influence the way of life, view of health and illness, and effectiveness of any health program.

It has been said repeatedly that better-educated people demand a higher level of health care. Knowledge of the educational level of a population is necessary if health services and programs are to be understood and accepted by the people and are to derive from their needs and desires. Comparison of educational levels of one community with another gives additional clues about the possible background of the people. There is a positive relationship between education and employment, housing, and socioeconomics in general.

Analysis of the proportion of families within certain income brackets and of the median income of families in a community can be very revealing in relation to a community's economics and employment patterns. Although high unemployment is often related to low educational levels and accompanying problems, there may be other national trends affecting the economy and contributing to unemployment. It is evident that an economically depressed community is not able to pay for quality care even if it be provided. The economic situation within a community has a great deal to do with establishment of priority of needs. For an economically depressed community, health may have the lowest priority and employment the highest.

The interrelationships between population characteristics such as age distribution, ethnicity, race, religion, education, income, and employment are integral and interdependent. Some of these have been identified. They will, however, take on more meaning when considered in relation to other aspects important to the life of a people, such as environment and patterns of health and illness.

Environmental Factors

The positive relationship between the environment and physical, social, and emotional health, though eminently clear, is seldom afforded the consideration which it deserves. A man is intimately and irrevocably dependent upon his environment. He can neither be separated from it nor viewed apart from it. He responds to it with every one of his senses. The environment encompasses a myriad of things, conditions, and situations which make up his very way of life.

Today's literature and other communication media are filled with expressions of concern about the ruthlessness and thoughtlessness with which man is destroying the beauty and usefulness of the land, polluting its rivers and streams, and poisoning the air and very food he eats. Environmental deterioration, the result of the composite of industrialization and technology, a rapidly expanding population, and a mobile urban society, gives justifiable cause for concern and is particularly significant to health workers.

Several key environmental factors, particularly significant to health, have been selected for analysis. They include housing, air, water, and sanitation, safety and protective measures, and finally transportation. Community health nursing must be alert to these and any additional environmental factors which might potentially have an adverse effect on health. Analysis of data about a community in which an airplane factory for example, is a key industry may suggest clues as to possible pollution and other health problems. Further exploration may either prove that there is a health hazard or may give evidence of the fact that adequate and careful health regulations are providing effective controls.

There is a direct relationship between health and housing. Therefore, analysis of data about the availability, adequacy, and acceptability of housing in a community gives clues about possible health hazards as well as socioeconomic status. For example, if analysis indicates that 50 percent of a community's housing is in fair to poor condition, and is occupied predominantly by blacks and Puerto Ricans, one can predict that health and health-related problems will differ from those of a neighboring middle-class suburb. The amount of crime and delinquency will be greater, accidents will be more frequent, and fires will occur more often. It can also be predicted, with certainty, that social and emotional problems associated with overcrowding and confusion will abound, and that infectious diseases, rat bites, and lead poisoning will occur with relatively high frequency. Analysis of these data suggests the need for a variety of protective, educative, and supportive services. It may also reveal such things as landlord exploitation of tenants, unsafe habitation, or failure of enforcement of existing housing codes and regulations. Community health nursing may need to become the advocate of the residents of the community for better living conditions.

Analysis of data concerning water supply, sanitation, sewerage, and trash disposal programs becomes particularly meaningful when viewed in relation to the concentration of population, its housing, and its needs. For example, if a particular housing development is expanding at such a rapid rate that sewerage, trash, garbage collection, and even a safe water supply are inadequate, there is obviously a potentially serious health problem. On the other hand, properly tested well water and cesspools may be perfectly safe and adequate for a rural community.

Protective services such as fire, police, civil defense, and safety must also be viewed in relationship to the population and its whole way of life. For example, in one very old section of a New England city, the streets (actually alleys) proved to be so narrow that it was impossible for fire equipment even to enter some of them. Residents of many of the apartments, which were inadequately heated, used space heaters—a practice which had serious consequences and resulted in devastating fires, burns, and poisoning from ingestion of kerosene. Fortunately, analysis of this data led health workers and concerned citizens to later select this area for urban redevelopment.

Analysis of the kind and frequency of accidents, assaults, and molestation of the population indicates the importance of gathering further data about such factors as how, where, and when the incidents occurred; what resources and facilities are available for prevention; what more are needed; and what are the best plans for future action.

In the first part of the book transportation was selected as one of the vital forces which contributed to the development of the country. Transportation is equally important to our way of life today. As might be expected, however, many of the current problems associated with it have changed.

Analysis of the kinds of transportation—trolley, bus, train, and automobile—and routes and patterns of transportation within and between communities gives health workers invaluable information as to how people can get to shops, to health facilities, to homes of other family members; how long travel to desired destinations takes and how many changes or transfers are necessary; what the expense of travel entails; how convenient the transportation is from place of residence to points of destination; and how well schedules are kept. Analysis of these and other pertinent data gives invaluable clues as to location of health resources, patterns of utilization of the services, and planning for different types and locations of future facilities. It provides the basis for consideration of the need for alternate kinds or sources of transportation.

The tension and even damage to hearing which can be caused by the roar and sonic boom of airplanes or the constant hum of superhighway traffic is often overlooked. Having information about situations of this kind in a community located adjacent to a large metropolitan airport can give some clues about possible physical or emotional problems.

Transportation is vital to our whole way of life. Mounting problems such as congestion, traffic jams, accidents, and air pollution, all associated with urbanization and all related to health, are demanding that community health nursing along with other health workers come up with new and innovative solutions.

Just as transportation is necessary for the movement of people and goods between and within communities, so is communication vital to a man's whole way of relating, learning, teaching, sharing, asking, helping, collaborating, and just living with and trying to understand his fellow man. Technologic and scientific developments have resulted in a proliferation of communication media such as television, radio, tape recorders, and telephones. Amounts and kinds of printed materials have also mushroomed. Analysis of the kinds of media which are available to a community, and how and to what extent they seem to be used, gives health workers clues as to how widely the population may have been exposed to health and health-related information in the past, and ideas about the communication resources appropriate for possible future health education and guidance programs.

Equally important is analysis of informal as well as formal sources of communication. Identification of individuals, groups, and organizations who tend to take leadership in either supporting or opposing community changes gives health workers better understanding of community dynamics. This adds to predictability of success or failure of future programs and gives a more realistic basis for the determination of how these key people can make their best contribution to the community and the advisability of their inclusion or representation on planning groups.

Health Information

Any meaningful health program must be planned in relation to the problems and needs of each community. These obviously cannot be identified until there has been careful analysis of data about the health of the people, their vital statistics, disease incidence and prevalence, and leading causes of death. Of importance are collection and analysis of additional data relative to unique problems of a particular community, such as one harboring an atomic plant or a coal mining industry.

Analysis of vital health statistics of a community parallels the medical history of a patient, or the analysis of health needs of a family in terms of its importance in determining a community's health. To illustrate, knowledge that the infant death rate of a community is 30.2 does not really pinpoint the factors which may account for this elevated rate. A look at the infant death rate of a community by census tracts, however, gives a much clearer picture. It may reveal that the rates in the two most heavily populated census tracts are 52.4 and 50.6, respectively. Further information may reveal that these are areas characterized by poor housing, considerable unemployment, and a high rate of illegitimacy; and also that two-thirds of the residents are either first or second generation foreign-born. These kinds of data all give clues about some of the socioeconomic and health-related problems and needs of mothers and children which may exist in this community and which should be investigated more definitively. They indicate the need for special services for prenatal patients, child health supervision, health guidance, and services for adolescents. The same "focusing in" process used in relation to the infant death rate can be applied to any other data about the community. It might well be used in relation to the maternal mortality rate in helping to determine the major factors which contribute to maternal mortality, and the implications for improved programs and services.

Analysis of the incidence and prevalence of heart disease, cancer, diabetes, and any other disease significant to a particular community must be carried out in relation to factors such as age distribution of the population, socioeconomic status, and resources and needs before valid clues basic to planning and priorities can be identified.

Analysis of the leading causes of death can be helpful in a variety of ways. For example, if the leading cause of death in one community is infectious disease, while that of the state or nation is heart disease, the implications for further exploration of sanitation, availability of preventive health programs, and adequacy of medical care and hospital facilities, as well as other facilities, are clear. On the other hand, if accidental death occurs frequently, data concerning the kinds and locations of accidents and the amount of disability resulting from them needs to be explored, as well as the community's resources for safety and for the prevention of health hazards. If one of the leading causes of death in a community is consistent with that of the state or the country, for example, heart disease, what are the resources and facilities for prevention, care, and rehabilitation for those with this particular health problem?

Inherent in the concept of comprehensive care is adequacy and quality of health resources, facilities, and personnel to make this a reality. Analysis of information about the hospitals, clinics, extended care facilities, and other health and health-related institutions will give clues not only to the adequacy of numbers and kinds of facilities, but also to their relationships to the health priorities of the people whom they serve. To illustrate, if in a community the incidence and prevalence of chronic disease are high, evaluation of the kinds of resources which are available to this group is specifically indicated. Analysis of health data about each segment of the population aids in determination of health problems, their priority, and possible solutions.

Just as vital statistics and health data give life and meaning to determination of health problems and needs in a community, so do health and health-related personnel give life and meaning to health facilities and resources. The growing army of professionals, professional assistants, specialists, consumers, neighborhood workers, and others has much to contribute to comprehensive care. To do this in any unified way, however, its members will have to learn better ways to communicate and to coordinate their efforts in order to avoid the fragmentation and confusion which now exists. Analysis of the kinds and numbers of personnel available to a community is necessary as no health program will succeed without enough sufficiently well-prepared personnel. Analysis of personnel resources also gives additional clues as to how various health workers might best contribute to a community—either by direct service, coordination, collaboration, or consultation.

Each category of data and information which community health nursing needs to have about a community with which it is concerned has been discussed and analyzed separately as to its significance to health. Some relationships have been identified and clues to possible health problems suggested. This first step in analysis is important. Analysis of these data becomes really meaningful when the total facts and information about each category are explored as a whole. A clearer, more unified picture comes into focus. Constellations of related factors and significant relationships emerge, and the relative priority of health in comparison with the other concerns of the people can be understood and defined. Identification of health problems is now possible.

A composite of the base-line data and their relationships provides the framework within which health problems and subsequent nursing needs of the community are derived. Just as beauty is in the eye of the beholder, so is the degree to which the significance of these data is meaningful related to the skill of the analyzer, in this instance community health nursing. In this process of analysis each professional group determines relationships and makes judgments based on its own knowledge, experience, and unique frame of reference.

A look first at population characteristics and health data of a community helps to pinpoint possible health problems. Health data, however, cannot be looked at in isolation. Throughout this chapter interrelationships between and among various characteristics of a community, its people, and their way of life and health have been pointed out and suggested as clues to identification of health problems. In essence the validity and effectiveness of this whole process of analysis rests with community health nursing's ability to understand the significance of these relationships, and to be able to identify the health problems which result.

The final extremely important step in analysis entails:

1. Looking at nursing services available to a community.
2. Looking at these nursing services in relation to the nursing needs which have been derived from the health problems.
3. Determining which of the needs nursing can or should do something about.

There are certain base-line data which nursing must have about the organizations and agencies currently providing community health nursing services within a particular community. These include kinds and extent of services provided; their availability, accessibility, and acceptability; comprehensiveness; utilization; costs; personnel; and finally the kinds and extent of relationships and patterns of inter-communication which have been established between and among agencies and personnel providing these services.

Community health nursing in one community may be provided by a one-nurse agency, and in another by a veritable patchwork of voluntary, official, and specialized agencies. A mass of data about any or all of these programs is meaningless until, as has been pointed out, it is analyzed in relation to the problems and needs of the people.

First, and extremely important, is consideration of the kinds of community health nursing services available to a community. Is there provision for bedside care of both the acute and chronically ill, for rehabilitation, prevention, and health promotion? The kinds of services provided may be comprehensive, but are they available for all age groups? For example, a hospital-based home care program may provide a gamut of hospital and home care services to its own patients, but what about others in the community who need care?

If the services are comprehensive and available to all age groups, are they accessible? Are they convenient to public transportation? The relationship between a community's transportation and the location of its health facilities will provide important information in answering questions about utilization of the services. If data indicate that 30 percent of the case load of the neighborhood clinic comes from another area of the city, how are the needs of the rest of the residents being met? What other factors might account for the fact that so few people take advantage of their own resources? Is the service acceptable to the people, or are there cultural or financial barriers which prevent maximum utilization? The relationship between utilization and the characteristics of the population contributes to further understanding of these factors.

The cost of care is a factor in influencing patterns of utilization. Information about the cost to the agency providing service, as well as the cost to the patient, often points out directions for exploration of other possible sources of financing. The cost to the patient must be analyzed in relationship to available third-party payments, such as Medicare, Medicaid, or Cancer Society, as well as to the socio-economic levels of the community in general.

Analysis of data about the personnel providing community health nursing services gives clues as to possible quantity, quality, and service patterns. If, for example, a large percentage of community health nurses in a particular community are experienced and educationally prepared, it can be assumed that the potential for quality of service is present. Additional information about such things as supervision, staff development, and team functioning gives further clues as to the possible extent and quality of the nursing program.

Study of the kinds of referrals and contractual agreements which have been developed between and among the nursing organizations gives clues about coordination of services and continuity of care. Additional information about community health nursing's participation on community planning groups adds another dimension to one's understanding of nursing's involvement in the community.

After analyzing the nursing services and resources available in a community, the next step is to study the relationship between these and the nursing needs which have been derived from the health problems. For example, in one community in which the majority of the residents are older retired persons, one of the major health problems might well be that of chronic disease. If analysis of the community health nursing services available to this population indicates that such services as bedside nursing in the home, rehabilitation, and extended care facilities are not adequately provided, but that the bulk of the nursing services of the community are for mothers and children, then it is evident that the nursing needs of this community are not being met. To illustrate further, it is more usual in a community where the maternal and child needs are the most pressing that the major emphasis of nursing service tends to be devoted to bedside nursing care of the sick. Further analysis of situations of this kind may well prove that the financial problems of an organization, coupled with the availability of income from federal sources, such as Medicare, have influenced the directions in which the programs have developed—and all too often, away from preventive and educative services. It must always be kept in mind that basic preventive and protective programs, such as those for tuberculosis and other communicable diseases, must always be maintained.

After the nursing services available to a community have been analyzed in relation to the nursing needs and health problems, community health nursing must decide which of these needs it can and should do something about. No individual or group can be all things to all people. Community health nursing, along with every other professional group, must be more discriminating and more skillful in setting priorities and limits as to what it can do, what it can do best, what it can help others to do, and what others can do better before more effective and comprehensive care will result.

When health problems of a community are those of chronic disease, infectious disease, or maternal and child health, for example, nursing obviously has an important and vital role to play in meeting its nursing needs. The health problems of greatest priority in another community, however, may be concern about an adequate water supply for an expanding population. This is of concern to community health nursing, but it is to the sanitary engineer that the community must turn for real solutions, and not to nursing. The health problem of yet another community may be drug addiction among teen-agers. In this instance, analysis of the number and variety of personnel in addition to community health nurses who are currently actively involved in developing a drug program within a community will help to pinpoint what and how community health nursing might best contribute. It may well be that there are several other high-priority health problems with more pressing nursing needs. Nursing may decide that in this instance it will not become actively involved with the drug problem but will work with others in a supportive and perhaps consultative role.

It is evident that even after nursing needs are determined, nursing cannot always meet all these needs, and must use its own best professional judgment in making decisions about priorities and future planning. This planning process, the basis for action, will be explored in the next chapter.

REFERENCES

American Public Health Association. A Self-Study Guide for Community Action-Planning, Vols. I and II. New York, American Public Health Association, 1967.

Duhl, L., ed. The Urban Condition. New York, Simon and Schuster, 1969.

Fox, J., Hall, C., and Elverback, L. Epidemiology: Man and Disease. New York, The Macmillan Company, 1970.

Hilleboe, H. E. Public health in the United States in the 1970's. Amer. J. Public Health, 58:1588-1610, September 1968.

Means, R. Interpreting statistics: An art. Nurs. Outlook, 13:34-37, May 1965.

National Commission On Community Health Services. Health Is a Community Affair. Cambridge, Mass., Harvard University Press, 1967.

Sparer, G., and Alderman, A. Data needs for planning neighborhood health centers. Amer. J. Public Health, 61:796-806, April 1971.

Stewart, D., and Vincent, P. Public Health Nursing. Dubuque, Iowa, William C. Brown Company, Publishers, 1968.

CHAPTER 13

Developing a Nursing
Plan of Action
for the Community

The discussion in this chapter focuses on the process through which community health nursing develops a plan of action to alleviate those aspects of a community's health problems which nursing can do something about—in other words, its nursing needs.

The process of planning is given the highest priority today. A new era of planning in America has been brought into sharp focus by many forces operating within its increasingly complex society: a national policy that health is a right of every individual; active participation of nonprofessionals on an expanding health team; greater knowledge of the direct relationship between illness and health; a national mandate for comprehensive health planning; new interest in and better technology for early detection of possible ills; emphasis on the needs of people rather than on agencies; and finally, realization that only through planning can something be done about the "wonderful and awful" health system which has evolved in America.

Planning is the basis for action, and this is an era of social action as well as planning. There is heightened awareness on the part of many who are.involved with health that only through the concerted and collaborative efforts of both health professionals and citizens throughout the land can this country begin to cope with its new and changing health hazards and utilize its resources for present and future health needs. Public health nurses from the beginning worked with the community and were concerned with its health. Today, however, this is a whole new ball game. Community health nursing is now part of a multifaceted health complex and is learning new ways to function in this expanding system. Its responsibility is greater than ever. It must take leadership in identifying nursing needs, interpreting them to others, participating in the planning and decision-making process, and helping to find new and innovative ways not only to provide nursing services but to develop the best mechanism by which these will reach those who need them—the consumers.

There are forces within community health nursing itself which make planning urgent: changing patterns for financing nursing care resulting from legislation such as Medicare; changing roles and responsibilities resulting from multipurpose patterns of nursing education and the expanding role of the nurse; proliferating health services which include community health nursing; the increasing amount of complex nursing care provided in the home; priority of comprehensiveness; and pressure from the consumer for better health care.

Further clarification of what is meant by planning and some of the principles basic to it, provide a background and frame of reference within which to look at the process. What does the word *planning* encompass? According to Mott:

> Planning is an effort on the part of some group or organization to alter the behavior and conditions of other people. No matter how objective or wise planners may be, they are engaged in deciding what is "good" for other people and taking steps to obtain that good.[1]

There are obviously pitfalls both in attempting to alter behavior of others and in making decisions which affect others. Planners have learned, many the hard way, that there are certain guidelines which are basic to sound planning and which contribute to the success of planning efforts. These are:

---

[1] Mott, B. J. The myth of planning without politics. *Amer. J. Public Health*, 59:797, May 1969.

1. Plans should be based on identified desires, needs, and interests of those for whom the plan is designed.

2. Those who will be involved in carrying out a plan should be involved in the planning.

3. Those who will have a major stake in the plan should be involved in planning.

4. The plan should be realistic in terms of people, money, and resources available; the best way to do the job; the best people to do the job; and the best chance of success possible.

Who should take the initiative in identifying the fact that something should be done about a community nursing need, for discussing this with others who are concerned, and helping to turn the wheels for action? More specifically, who is responsible for initiating community health nursing planning? It is clearly the responsibility of the community health nurse since the community is her patient. However, she has not always assumed leadership but has all too often sat back and waited for someone else to take the initiative. Too often the needs of an agency or a particular geographic area have been the focus for action. Too often nurses in key positions within the community have exerted influence in relation to their own agency's program and vested interest, without necessarily taking into consideration the nursing needs of the broader community. This does not suggest that the total responsibility for planning community health nursing rests with nursing and nursing alone. The task of planning is too important and too big to leave entirely to nurses. It also demands the best thinking, resources, and skills of many others. Nursing, however, has primary responsibility for seeing that the nursing needs of the community are met. It must determine what it can do best, and when it needs to call on others for assistance and guidance.

For purposes of clarification, the process of developing a plan of action to meet the nursing needs of the community is presented here as a series of separate and consecutive steps. This is done with full realization that there is some danger in this segmental approach, since in reality the steps are interrelated and often interchangeable. These steps are:

1. Preplanning to meet the identified nursing needs.

2. Determining the desired goal or goals to alleviate the nursing need.

3. Evaluating the alternative choices for reaching the goals.

4. Establishing short and long range goals.
5. Choosing the best course of action to reach these goals.

Each of these steps will be explored separately.

Preplanning to Meet the Identified Nursing Needs

The need for preplanning, as well as its value, has become increasingly evident in such a complex society as ours. It provides opportunity for decision making about who should be involved in planning, and for determination of the parameters or limits within which a plan is to be developed. In other words, some preliminary decisions are made at this time, and the stage is set for more effective planning.

Community health nursing needs to ask itself first, who should be involved in developing the plan of action? Should nursing do this alone or in conjunction with others? It is obvious that there is no one answer to these questions. It may be most appropriate, in some instances, for nursing to solve its own problems. In others, it may need help. The nature and extent of the nursing needs, and the size and complexity of the community and its health problems will help to determine the kind and number of planners who should be involved. Consideration needs to be given to the inclusion and or representation in some aspect of the planning of:

1. Those for whom the plan is designed, the consumer. In the final analysis, he, like community health nursing, has his own area of expertise. He is the one who can best interpret the desires, interests, and needs of the public. The final decision about community action rests with him.

2. Those who are concerned with the problem. Among those who share in formulation of plans for its solution should be included professionals and other health-related groups who are concerned with the community.

3. Those who appear best able to contribute to planning by virtue of ability, position, knowledge, or experience.

4. Those (community health nurses and others) who are most likely to follow through in carrying out a plan by virtue of interest, power, or motivation.

Many other members of the health team and the community, as

well as nurses, have a vital stake in nursing and a valuable contribution to make to the solution of its problems. The primary responsibility of nursing, however, still rests with nursing—just as the ultimate success of community action rests with the citizen for whom it exists.

Any planning group, no matter how well selected or representative, can be so large that it becomes unwieldy and unproductive. Everyone concerned with the problem cannot personally be represented in its alleviation, but the interests of those who are concerned can and must be considered in the deliberations. This can be done best by the inclusion in planning of representatives who are acceptable to those whom they represent and qualified to speak for them. Others can be added or consulted whenever this seems desirable. Community health nursing may hold several preliminary discussions with key people before actually deciding who will become directly involved in planning.

Preplanning also provides opportunity for community health nursing to study the relationship between the community's nursing needs and the priorities of its health problems, and to determine priorities among the nursing needs for which the plan of action is being developed. This helps to keep needs and goals in proper focus and further ensures that the contribution and efforts of nursing will be directed toward solutions of the health problems of a community.

Determining the Nursing Goals

The ultimate goals for alleviation of the existing nursing needs of a community give purpose and direction, and provide a focal point for the planning effort. Since these goals are the targets for action, they should be clearly understood and viewed as desirable and realistic by the planning group. In setting goals, community health nursing must take leadership in determining the kinds and priorities of nursing services which will best meet the needs of the community. The goals, to be realistic, must focus on the nursing aspects of the three broad components of a community's health—health maintenance, health promotion, and disease prevention. If, for example, health maintenance receives the lion's share of attention and effort in a community, and prevention is neglected, the ultimate effect on the level of immunization and other disease prevention programs could well be disastrous.

There may be one goal or several goals toward which action is to be directed. For example, let us assume that the health problem of highest priority in one particular community, determined on the basis of all the data, was found to be in the maternal and child area, that nursing services, resources, and facilities for mothers and children were also inadequate, and that a whole constellation of nursing needs was identified. In such a situation the specificity and clarity with which community health nursing states its desired goals for mothers and children can make a great deal of difference to planning. Too often the goal is stated as the much to be desired but seldom attained "comprehensive health care for mothers and children." One cannot deny that this is exemplary. It would be just as heretical to be against comprehensive care as against motherhood itself, but it is like the pot of gold at the end of the rainbow, hard to reach. The fact is that such an abstract, nonspecific, all-inclusive goal does little to point out to those attempting to attain it the best road for them to follow. Equally important, how can one measure or evaluate specific progress toward such a diffuse goal? The point to be made here is that goals need to be stated in clear, measurable, behavioral terms which in turn can serve as measuring rods for progress toward attainment. Community health nursing, therefore, should carefully determine what it wishes to do to specifically alleviate the nursing needs of mothers and children in the community. Some of the goals might be stated as follows:

> All high-risk pregnant women will receive nursing supervision.
>
> Private physicians and clinics providing maternity services will refer all these women for nursing supervision.
>
> All premature infants will receive home nursing supervision.
>
> The number of expectant parents attending group classes will increase by 50 percent.

These are only a few of the nursing goals in the maternal and child health program. They do, however, illustrate the point being made. Each goal is stated in relation to the behavior that can be observed and measured, and gives definite direction to those developing a plan of action.

The fact that any plan for a community must be viewed as valuable by the consumer has been noted many times throughout this book. Therefore, the goals toward which action is directed must first and foremost be acceptable to the community, as well as being clearly defined and measurable.

Evaluating Alternative Choices for Reaching the Goals Inherent in this step of the planning process is recognition that there are many factors operating within a community which can influence planning either positively or negatively. Some of the factors which may affect the success or failure of a plan are: possible barriers to community change, such as vested interests, traditions, patterns of organization, and finances; forces within the community such as politics and power; factors such as previous experience and timing; and contemporary concepts related to planning, such as community of solution and regionalization.

It is one thing to spell out the steps in planning for community health nursing, and another to carry them out in today's complex, changing, and, to date, unclear situation. One is tempted to look back on the pattern of yesterday's community health nursing service with a certain nostalgia. It seemed so simple, with the major portion of public health nursing services provided by either the official or voluntary nursing program. In reality, it was almost monopolistic. Basic responsibilities were spelled out for the official agency. The voluntary nursing agencies, for the most part, decided what services they would provide, determined their costs, and decided whom they would employ. Exclusive of those public health nursing programs which were generalized or combined, lines of demarcation between the official and voluntary programs were quite clearly understood. Although it would be presumptuous to claim that those traditional services were consistently of the best quality, or inclusive, there was in most communities a recognizable, discernible network of community health nursing services. There is little relationship between the situation of yesterday and that of today in most communities, particularly in metropolitan areas. New and different services, both comprehensive and specialized, are provided by satellite clinics, neighborhood centers, and model cities programs, to name a few. Some of these have carved out islands of special services for selected groups and have left gaps and holes in a former, though perhaps thin, community nursing fabric. The agencies which traditionally provided most of these services have adjusted to the changes in a variety of ways. In some instances they have taken leadership in the development of new and innovative programs. In others, through contractual agreements, they have provided staff or services to a variety of programs. It must be recognized that the health market today is competitive in terms of patterns of service and organization, as well as manpower. There is also competition in relation to finances. Revenue from United Funds, traditionally an important source of income for many voluntary nursing agencies, is less abundant today. Increasingly, a larger proportion of this source of income is directed toward the needs of ghetto areas. This trend is of grave concern to suburban communities and is causing them real financial problems and worries. It is true that there are additional sources of income through federal programs such as Medicare and the Poverty Program which pay for a growing amount of care. Federal financing, however, influences the direction and emphasis of the programs which provide these kinds of care. It must be recognized that there are almost as many vested interests as there are programs providing community health nursing services, and at present there is very little agreement about just what the most desirable pattern for the future ought to be. All these factors influence and affect any planning relative to community health nursing. Any planning group, no matter how representative, will need to come to grips with the relationship between these vested interests and what is best ultimately for the greatest number of people within the community—for the consumer and not the agency. Therefore, vested interests and traditions, as well as patterns of organization and financing, can be barriers to change and can influence planning.

There are other factors which must be taken into consideration by those planning community health nursing services. One of these is politics—politics in the sense of how a group arrives at what is best for it, its goals. This kind of politics includes the efforts of the planners, as individuals and representatives of organizations, to utilize their skill, power, and persuasiveness to obtain their desired goals. This takes not only leadership but also cooperation and willingness to arbitrate. It also demands flexibility and real interest in a common goal.

Closely allied to politics is power. Every system within a community has its power structure, and community health nursing is no exception. The larger, or richer, or more prestigious community health nursing agencies have usually had the most power in decision making, and have often used this in the community through informal decisions made by relatively few people. Prestige is power and so is money. The source of a great deal of new money for community health nursing services today is the federal government. The federal government is big power, but the federal system at the present time is not really designed for partnership. The extent to which community health nursing programs within a community are dependent upon federal funds and regulations is a factor of growing importance today and one which must be reckoned with in any community planning. In the end, every community must work out its own community health nursing program to fit its own politics and power, its own special problems and resources, and its own community personality.

Community health nurses involved in planning must carefully consider the timing for any plan of action. Timing may be the key factor in the success or failure of any plan. Improper timing may result in apathy or strong resistance to any suggestion, resistance due in reality to factors unrelated to community health nursing. For example, the community may have just been through a period of rapid change and upheaval by virtue of a massive redevelopment program. It may need to regain its equilibrium before tackling further problems. Conversely, acceptance of a plan may be made easier because a particular community is interested and ready for change and accepts social action and progress as valuable. The priority which the community places on a particular problem at a particular time is part of the picture. Sensitivity to the pulse of the community, therefore, is of the essence for community health nursing. Closely related to timing are the past experiences of a community and the ways in which it has previously responded to change. Also important are the composition of the community, the extent of involvement of its citizens in community affairs, and the relationships which have been developed.

It must always be kept in mind that any community, big or small, is part of a larger society and must be looked at within this context. The ways in which contemporary society views health problems, and the kinds of approaches it is using for their solutions have a real impact on community planning for nursing. There are two concepts in particular which should be considered. They are "community of solution" and "regionalization."

As previously pointed out, no individual community can or necessarily should provide all its own health services, resources, or facilities. It cannot, likewise, find solutions for all the problems within its own boundaries. The National Commission on Community Health Services suggests:

that where health services are concerned the boundaries of each community are established by the boundaries within which a problem can be defined, dealt with, and solved.[2]

And further that:

As the center of responsibility for assuring that personal and environmental health services are available to all residents, the community should first assay its resources, its programs and needs, and the strengths that exist to meet these needs. After the community has assessed its resources, it can join with other communities to solve larger problems that require resources of a larger geographic region, a wider political jurisdiction, and more funding than is available to one locality.[3]

This concept of the community of solution is of the utmost importance to community health nursing planners. The needs of a mobile population are constantly changing, and each new problem must be studied in relation to the particular boundaries within which it can be solved. For example, a community's need for home health services may be far better met by arrangements through a contractual agreement to purchase this from a large, well-established neighborhood agency, rather than establishing its own. This concept can also be applied to better utilization of the larger health team.

Closely related to the concept of community of solution is that of regionalization. Although each community is unique, adjoining communities or areas have many common interests, as well as problems. It is reasonable that planning for health services within geographic regions having similar interests and problems makes possible better use and distribution of these resources, facilities, and money. The federal government gave little direct encouragement to regional planning for health until 1966 when the 89th Congress passed the Regional Medical Programs Act and the Comprehensive Health Planning Act.

There is heightened interest in regionalization and the utilization of this concept in planning. Many community health nurses, as well as other health workers, know that regional planning for health services is paramount and will come about some day. Questions and fears are being raised about who will control these regional community health nursing services, who will be left out, and what the implication will be for official and voluntary nursing services alike.

[2]National Commission on Community Health Services. *Health Is a Community Affair.* Cambridge, Mass., Harvard University Press, 1967, p. 2.
[3]*Ibid.,* p. 4.

These factors—barriers to change, community forces, previous experience and timing and contemporary concepts—must be kept in mind by community health nursing as it studies and evaluates the totality of information it has about a community, in order to determine the best and most realistic plan of action to meet its individual nursing needs. Just as vital statistics, health, and population data help to pinpoint health problems, so do certain other characteristics of a community give community health nursing clues about the feasibility, acceptability, and predictable success of a possible plan of action. These data, which include communication, socioeconomics, education, environment, population, resources, facilities, and finances, cannot be viewed apart from their interrelationships with the community and the nursing needs being considered. The same kinds of data are valuable to many health workers. However, the way in which community health nursing interprets their value and meaning in relation to the health needs of the community is the uniqueness of nursing.

Evaluation of alternative courses for reaching the desired goal or goals demands the very best skill and professional judgment of community health nursing. It involves making decisions, proposing, and choosing alternative plans of action. In this process community health nursing must:

1. Identify the key factors which may account for a nursing need.
2. Study these in relation to the totality of knowledge and information which it has about the community.
3. Consider the feasibility of alternate plans of action.
4. Make choices and decisions about the future course of action.

The following illustration will help to clarify the steps by which community health nursing decides on a plan of action in relation to one of the nursing goals which it has established for a community. The goal was stated as, "All high-risk pregnant women will receive nursing supervision."

Classification of who comprises this high-risk group must be clearly understood and acceptable to the planners in order to avoid possible confusion and misunderstanding. What are some of the key factors which may account for this nursing need and prevent high-risk pregnant women from receiving nursing supervision? Are there enough facilities? Are they conveniently located? Are they utilized? Do the pregnant women know about the services which are available?

Who refers them for nursing supervision? Do they view these services as valuable? Are there enough nursing personnel in the community to provide supervision? Are the nursing personnel adequately prepared? Are there enough financial resources? Are there problems unique to certain categories of these pregnant women?

Some key factors, identified on the basis of the foregoing questions, which account for this nursing need might be: lack of knowledge on the part of these women about either the value or availability of nursing supervision; few referrals from hospitals or other health resources; and minimal amount of nursing supervision provided in the areas with the greatest amount of need.

These are some of the factors which may prevent many high-risk pregnant women from receiving nursing supervision. Each needs to be carefully studied in relation to the community. What might account for the fact that these women do not know about the value or availability of nursing supervision? What are the patterns of communication within this community? How might people get this kind of information? What is the educational level? What are the cultural patterns and attitudes toward health? What are the sources of health information? Is there an interagency referral system? What value do other health workers who might refer these women or inform them about nursing supervision place on this kind of care? What are the resources or mechanisms by which high-risk women might be better informed about the value and availability of nursing supervision?

After these factors have been identified and studied, consideration must be given to alternative plans of action. Some possible considerations might be to:

1. Develop a health education program within the community which would hopefully reach this group of patients.

2. Plan a staff development program or workshop for community health nursing and other key health workers involved with these patients.

3. Organize and inform neighborhood aides in high-risk neighborhoods.

4. Develop an interagency referral system involving individuals, groups, and institutions concerned with this group of women.

5. Strengthen the sex education and health counseling programs within the junior high and the high school.

Priorities need to be developed for these possible alternative choices of action in order to determine which plan or combination of plans has the greatest chance of being the most effective and efficient in the light of the particular community and its totality of resources.

Establishing Short- and Long-Term Goals

Equally as important as determining a plan of action is the establishment of short-and long-range goals. This is necessary for several reasons. Some of these are:

1. Short-term goals serve the very important function of providing opportunity for responsiveness to the immediate and felt needs of the community and in addition constitute steps toward long-term goals. Long-term goals provide the focus which keeps planning headed in the direction of the improvement of a community's health.

2. One step toward a goal often depends upon another. Thus, long-term goals are often based on the series of short-term goals. For example, an older multipara woman may not be able to avail herself of nursing supervision because there are no day-care facilities available for the care of her children. Establishment of day-care centers first will remove one of the barriers to this problem.

3. Establishment of a series of short-term goals gives community health nursing the opportunity to try out or experiment with different mechanisms for change, evaluate and measure their effectiveness concerning progress toward a long-term goal, and make any changes necessary for future plans of action. For example, if the long-range goal for the future pattern of organization of nursing within a community is generalization of services, one short-term goal might be to experiment first with combining services in just one area of a community. An evaluation of this goal will determine how generalization of the remainder of the services might best be accomplished.

4. Community health nursing is concerned about the health of the community and the need to provide necessary nursing services. It is easier to measure progress toward a short-term than a long-term goal. Evidence of progress gives planners a sense of accomplishment and satisfaction. It serves as a basis for future planning and contributes an added factor of positive motivation to the planners.

In establishing both short- and long-range goals, community health nursing must always keep in mind that nursing needs are only one part of a whole constellation of a community's other needs, and must be viewed in this context if they are to have any predictable chance for success.

Choosing the Course of Action   After short- and long-range goals have been established, the next step in the planning process is choosing the best course of action to meet these goals. The difficulty in separating the steps of the planning process is evident, and a great deal of overlapping exists between the establishment of goals and deciding on ways in which they might best be reached. Although short- and long-term goals suggest directions for action, they do not designate the specific course of action. There are almost always several ways to get from one point to another. Considering alternatives and selecting the best way to reach the desired goal demands judgment based on knowledge, as well as creativity and imagination. For example, if development of an interagency referral system within a community is the goal of community health nursing, what is the best way to make this a reality? Would it be better for community health nursing to plan a workshop on referral for key people from all the agencies within the community who might be involved? Or would it be better to have a series of meetings with key people from each agency within the community? Or would it be better to meet with doctors, social workers, nurses, and others in individual groups? Or would it be better to try and develop a referral system between two agencies, evaluate the results, and then decide on next steps?

Different courses of goal-directed action must be considered and evaluated, and choices made in the light of each community's uniqueness and totality. The community itself, in the final analysis, holds the key to the success or failure of any plan of action.

In this chapter the process of planning to meet the nursing needs of the community has been explored and discussed. A plan, to be successful, must be realistic and clearly thought out as to goals, methods of accomplishment, and measurement. Equally important, it must be acceptable to the consumer and consistent with his whole way of life and his constellation of needs if it is to fulfill its purpose. Harnish aptly sums up the importance of planning when he says:

We have come to a point in America where the atmosphere for planning has been built. But until such a time as our personal involvement in this process proves that giving up one's autonomy and that of one's organization in cooperative action is rewarding and self-fulfilling, we shall not make full use of the great potential found in the health professions of America for creating truly healthy communities.[4]

How well community health nursing can capture this essence of planning is a sign of its true professionalism.

Implementation and evaluation of a plan are equally as important as its development. These are discussed in Chapter 14.

REFERENCES

Conant, R. W. The Politics of Community Health. National Commission on Community Health Services, Report of the Community Action Studies Project. Washington, D. C., Public Affairs Press, 1968.

Freeman, H. E., Levine, S., and Reeder, L. Handbook of Medical Sociology. Englewood Cliffs, N. J., Prentice-Hall, Inc., 1963.

Freeman, R. B. Community Health Nursing Practice. Philadelphia, W. B. Saunders Company, 1970.

Fifer, E. Z. Hangups in health planning. Amer. J. Public Health, 59:765-769, May 1969.

Fonaroff, A. Identifying and developing health services in a new town. Amer. J. Public Health, 60:821-828, May 1970.

Griffith, E. I. Where do the VNA's go from here? Nurs. Outlook, 16:29-31, March 1968.

Harnish, T. I. Regional medical program planning. Amer. J. Public Health, 59: 770-772, May 1969.

Henkel, B. O. Community Health. Boston, Allyn and Bacon, Inc., 1970.

Hilleboe, H. E. Editorial. Concepts of comprehensive health planning. Amer. J. Public Health, 58:1011-1013, June 1968.

Lewis, C. E. The thermodynamics of regional planning. Amer. J. Public Health, 59:773-777, May 1969.

Mattison, B. F. Community health planning and the health professions. Amer. J. Public Health, 58:1015-1021, June 1968.

Mott, B. F. The myth of planning without politics. Amer. J. Public Health, 59:797-803, May 1969.

National Commission on Community Health Services. Health Is A Community Affair. Cambridge, Mass., Harvard University Press, 1967.

Polk, L. D. Areawide comprehensive health planning: The Philadelphia story. Amer. J. Public Health, 59:760-764, May 1969.

Sanders, I. T. The Community. New York, The Ronald Press Company, 1958.

Sheahan, M. W. Through community action: A health commission reports. Amer. J. Nurs., 66:1298-1302, June 1966.

Silver, G. A. What Has Been Learned About the Delivery of Health Services to the Ghetto? In Norman, J. C., ed., Medicine in the Ghetto. New York, Appleton-Century-Crofts, 1969, pp. 65-72.

[4]Harnish, T. I. Regional medical program planning. *Amer. J. Public Health*, 59:772, May 1969.

CHAPTER 14

Implementing and Evaluating a Nursing Plan of Action for the Community

The final steps in the process by which community health nursing works with the community as the patient are implementation and evaluation of a nursing plan of action. Each of these steps will be discussed separately.

Implementation of a Nursing Plan of Action

Implementation of a plan for nursing within the community involves mobilization for action of existing identified resources (people, facilities, services, and money) in better or different ways to reach desired or identified goals. Implementation, to be sound, must be based on a plan or blueprint for action which has goals and priorities related to identified needs—in this instance nursing needs. Chapters 10 through 13 have been concerned with discussion of the components which are basic to the development of this blueprint. Since the planning process is a continuum, the difficulty in discussing a plan of action and its implementation separately is obvious. Aspects of planning which were mentioned previously will be more fully explored in this chapter.

Some general discussion of implementation will give a frame of reference within which to look at how community health nursing carries out a plan of action for nursing. Implementation carries with it grave responsibility and is one of the most strategic parts of the whole planning process. Its very purpose is to bring into being a different and improved product, in this instance nursing. Change is one of its inherent and inescapable ingredients: change in the kind and organization of nursing services for the community; change in the role and responsibilities of nursing and other personnel; and change in the allocation of funds for nursing. Change can be threatening and anxiety-producing, as well as exciting and rewarding. It must always be kept in mind that those who are most directly affected by change are more willing to change when they see the ultimate goal as desirable and consistent with their own value systems and interests. Community health nursing, therefore, must be sensitive to these dynamics of change, and skillful in basing judgment on broad knowledge of the characteristics and nursing needs of each community, whatever its size, composition, or complexity. Implementation demands not only sound judgment but also imagination and resourcefulness. It provides unlimited opportunities for innovation and creativity within a framework of reality. The sky may not always be the limit, but there are almost always ways to raise the ceiling. Flexibility is another ingredient of implementation. A course of action may need to be redirected or revised as a result of additional clues, inappropriate timing, new knowledge, new research or evaluation. Implementation, however, demands commitment to priority and goals as well as flexibility.

Action toward the alleviation of one nursing need may result in other new and unanticipated problems. Medicare is a good case in point. This legislation, which was a response on the part of the federal government to the health needs of the elderly, has made possible and available better care for greater numbers of this segment of the population. The Medicare program, however, has had a profound effect on home health agencies—many of which now give greater priority to the care of the sick than to disease prevention and health promotion. The real skill in this whole planning process rests with the ability of the planner to respond to the myriad of real and immediate needs and demands of the community while also keeping in mind priorities and working toward long-term goals. Each community must study its own situation and decide how it can best mobilize and utilize its resources to reach its goals while, at the same time, responding to today's urgent need for immediate, better, and different health services.

Some of the base-line data about the community such as resources, facilities and services, finances, socioeconomics, transportation, and dynamics have particular relevance for implementation, but must be viewed in relation to all aspects of the community.

The process of implementation includes the following steps:

1. Ascertaining resources
2. Mobilizing resources
3. Activating the plan

The process of implementation presented in this chapter is not exclusive to community health nursing, but the way nursing applies the process for action is unique. Many other health workers are attempting to reach the same broad comprehensive goals for the health of the community as is community health nursing. Proliferation of knowledge and of specialists has demanded that several people concerned with a common problem pool their resources and expertise and work together for its solution. Increasingly, health workers are using this approach. It must be recognized that there are gray, unclear areas of responsibility and that there is overlapping of function. There is also considerable role confusion among many health workers with resulting inefficient utilization of resources, particularly scarce and precious human resources, and fragmentation of service. The term multidiscipline presupposes that each discipline is different and has a unique contribution to make to the whole. One main purpose of this book is to clarify the process of community health nursing. This is done with full realization that nursing has membership on an expanding health team and does not do the job alone. It must, however, be clear about each step of the nursing process in order to contribute its unique professional expertise to the broader health team.

Ascertaining Resources   The first step in implementa-
                                     tion is to ascertain which re-
                                     sources are appropriate for the
                                     anticipated   nursing   action.
With the blueprint for nursing action in hand, community health
nursing must look at the base-line information about nursing facilities and services, resources, and money in relation to its relevance
and implication for the implementation of the desired nursing action.
First, a look at facilites and services. Just as the health care system is
complex, dynamic, and changing, so is the nursing care system within
it. The fragmentation, instability, and individuality of contemporary
nursing services makes it unrealistic and even impossible at this time
to suggest one best or most desirable nursing pattern. In reality there
are almost as many patterns as there are communities, and no one of
them is ideal. Community health nursing, therefore, when implementing a nursing plan, must look carefully at the network of
services which make up the nursing delivery care system within a
particular community. It must be aware of the fact that nursing
services are provided by various groups and under various auspices,
that some of the nursing personnel providing these services are well
prepared professionally and some are not, and that part of the
services are provided under the auspices of organized nursing and
part are under other auspices. One must be alert to what is going on
in nursing within the community.

Nursing services may be provided by one or a combination of
organizations. The patterns of community health nursing service
most familiar are those provided by voluntary and official agencies.
The visiting nurse association, a voluntary organization, is primarily a
nursing agency. The major thrust of its program is to provide nursing
care on a part-time basis to individuals who are sick in their own
homes. In providing services to the individuals who are sick, the
health and nursing needs of the entire family are taken into consideration with prevention of disease, promotion of health, and health
teaching an inherent part of the program. However, first priority for
service is usually the bedside nursing needs of individuals.

The health department, an official agency, is organized according
to the governmental structure of the local area. Thus, we find county
health departments, city health departments, metropolitan health
departments, and health departments for a single town or township.
The community health nursing program is just one of several programs of the health department. More than half of the budgeted

positions are for nurses. The major responsibilities of the nursing program within the health department are prevention and control of disease, health promotion, and health teaching for all groups. The activities of the nurse to carry out these responsibilities vary according to local conditions and facilities. Many of her activities consist of participation in clinics of various kinds, such as tuberculosis, well-child conferences, immunizations, multiphasic screening, mental retardation, antepartum, and postpartum. School nursing may also be her responsibility in some communities. Home visits are an integral part of these activities. Bedside nursing is not considered one of the major functions, but there is a trend toward the nursing program in health departments becoming certified as a Home Health Agency. The services of the health department and visiting nurse association may be provided separately, may be combined, or generalized.

Although a sizable proportion of nursing service continues to be provided by these agencies with which we are more familiar, a growing proportion is provided by an increasing array of new and different kinds of agencies and organizations. Many hospitals have extended their health services out into the community, and through home care programs and satellite clinics are attempting to meet its health needs. Some of these services are offered to specific groups such as mothers or children, and some are for specific areas of the community. Categorical federal legislation, such as that for heart, cancer, and stroke or for certain age groups, has resulted in a proliferation of special programs for selected persons. Attempts are being made to meet the multiple needs of people through multiservice centers, neighborhood centers, model cities programs, or prepaid group insurance plans, to name a few. Many of these multiple needs are for nursing. There are other new and exciting attempts to provide health care to the community through storefront clinics, mobile clinics, traveling vans, and family life centers.

Community health nursing is involved in this kaleidoscope of programs in a variety of ways. The task of dissecting out the fabric of the nursing care system from this crazy quilt for closer scrutiny is difficult. It must be done, however, before additional nursing action is attempted, as purposeless or unwise action may further compound the confusion which already exists.

The nursing care system does not exist apart from the people who give it life and meaning—nurses and the growing army of nursing and health-related workers. Community health nursing must ascertain which personnel will be most helpful and effective in contributing to and carrying out a nursing plan of action. Most of this information has already been collected, but again needs to be further scrutinized. First, what about community health nurses? How many nurses, both active and retired, are available to a community? What is their educational preparation and experience? How many are clinical specialists? How many licensed practical nurses, home health aides, and nursing aides are there? How are these nursing and nursing-related personnel currently being utilized within the community? Are there nursing or multidiscipline teams in operation? What about nursing coordinators? What other kinds of personnel besides nurses—doctors, doctors' assistants, social workers, consumers, and others—might contribute to the community?

A nursing care system, to be viable, must have adequately prepared personnel. It must also have money. Information about the current financial resources available to a community for nursing is extremely important. In addition to federal monies for the variety of programs previously mentioned, what about other available financial sources for nursing: grants, United Fund, Blue Cross, Blue Shield, Easter Seal, and other third-party payments? On the basis of all this information community health nursing decides which of these resources should most appropriately be involved in the anticipated nursing action.

Mobilizing the Resources

The second step is mobilization of these resources for effective nursing action. Which people can do the job best? What facilities or agencies should be involved? What money is available? How can mobilization be accomplished? Nursing must take leadership in selecting, channeling, and directing the resources for nursing action. The question of how this is to be done is of the essence. It is not always easy to spot the key people in the community who are most appropriate for the task at hand. Every community has its leaders, both professional and lay. It is important to identify them, to enlist their help, and gain their sanction and support. They may exert considerable influence and power because of politics, or money, or position and can often contribute to the success or failure of a plan of action. Who in the community has the best experience and background for the task at hand? Who is appropriate, acceptable, and above all, interested and concerned about the actions being planned? Every community has an untapped and limitless reservoir of human potential from which to draw. The consumer also has much to contribute. He knows what he wants and is learning how best and where to get it. He is highly motivated toward goals which he understands and values. He wants to participate and must be included. Care must be taken, however, to identify the consumer who really speaks for and represents the people. Community health nursing must also learn to recognize and utilize the contribution of the growing army of paraprofessionals. Failure to include them appropriately in nursing action may result in further duplication and fragmentation of service.

Mobilization of the resources of agencies and organizations, as well as people, involves knowledge of power and politics, vested interests, and finances. It is not an easy task. Every community, however, has a wealth of untapped resources, both human and material, and a boundless supply of ingenuity.

Some of the methods or mechanisms which further mobilization are communication, collaboration, and coordination. Communication is the bridge by which people understand each other, teach, learn, and share ideas. Those who are involved in any action or venture want to know what is going on and want to be kept informed. Channels of communication among all who are to be involved in nursing action must be kept open. Collaboration means working or laboring together toward a common goal—nursing action. Coordination is the harmonious interaction of those equal in rank or importance. Coordination, therefore, unifies. Both collaboration and coordination necessitate mutual respect and understanding, and a willingness to seek and give help. They mean free channels of communication, continuous dialogue, and a commitment to work together for what is best for the community. It is through effective communication, collaboration, and coordination that people and facilities are helped to mobilize effectively for nursing action.

Activating the Nursing Plan

The last and most important step in implementation is activating the plan—the end toward which the entire planning process has been directed. Community health nursing must be creative, willing to try out different approaches, and eager to experiment in trying to find better ways to use its knowledge and resources to serve the community. Two ways by which improved nursing services might be offered are: developing a new program; augmenting or expanding an existing program. Each possible plan of action must be critically evaluated as to its appropriateness and soundness. To illustrate, let us assume that more adequate nursing supervision for unmarried, pregnant, adolescent girls must be provided in a particular community. Some of the ways in which this might be accomplished are:

1. Establish a new satellite clinic for nursing supervision of this group of pregnant girls. Is this plan realistic in terms of personnel, facilities, and funds? Will the nursing staff for this satellite clinic have to be drawn from other nursing programs within the community? If so, what about the other nursing services? Is a specialized clinic desirable? Would this group of pregnant girls utilize a specialized clinic? Would the community accept this kind of a clinic?

2. Augment the nursing staff and resources of the agencies currently providing maternity care in the community in order that adequate services will be available for this group of pregnant women. How would these services be augmented? Should only the staff of the clinic in the geographic area of greatest need be augmented, or those of all the clinics and services in the community? Would additional or better-prepared staff be needed? Would a staff development program be advisable?

3. Develop a health counseling and guidance program within the junior high and high school, and a referral system between these schools and the agencies currently providing nursing supervision to maternity patients. Can the health counseling and guidance program within the junior and high school be expanded, or must a new program be developed? Will the school personnel and parents accept such a program? Will the students utilize it? How would referrals be made?

4. Organize a group of adolescent girls within the community and work with them in planning both discussion groups for teen-agers and a drop-in center for information and referral. Should the drop-in center be for multiproblem information and referral rather than for this one special problem? How might the community accept this drop-in center? Would teen-agers be apt to utilize it?

Community health nursing must decide in each particular community whether any one of these proposed plans might be realistic, acceptable, or even feasible in the light of the total situation. It must also keep in mind such things as current practices and trends, regional patterns, and the area in which the problem can best be solved—the community of solution. It must ask itself the important question in relation to any program change: Will improvement in one aspect of a program result in deterioration of another? It must also keep in mind that legislation, such as a national health insurance plan, will of necessity markedly affect any and all community planning for nursing, as well as other aspects of health.

Mention should be made of two of the mechanisms commonly used for coordination of nursing action within the community, contractual agreements and interagency referrals. It is often possible, through contractual agreements, for one agency or community to buy or obtain service from another, thus allowing for better use and distribution of personnel. Likewise, interagency referrals provide a whole network for the sharing of information and responsibilities between agencies and personnel and result in a more continuous and effective pattern of nursing within the community.

There are also other ways to bring about nursing action. For example, community health nursing might organize a central registry for community health nurses, so that the supply of nurses with particular preparation or experience would be more readily available and evenly distributed. In this way it would be less necessary to "rob Peter to pay Paul." Another community might organize and employ a community health nursing coordinator for the community, to ensure that the nursing needs of the community and not the needs of the agencies would be the focus for action. This community coordinator might well be a community health nursing specialist. Another community might establish a coordinating council composed of representatives from all organized nursing in the community, including hospitals, nursing homes, schools, industry, health departments, visiting nurse associations, and other organizations. In still another, they might establish a coordinating council composed of both nurses and consumers.

Community health nursing must always keep in mind that change or action in any part of the nursing system affects the whole system, and that there are administrative considerations which cannot be overlooked. The overall purpose of administration in any organization is to provide the structure or framework within which personnel can organize to accomplish the job to be done as effectively and efficiently as possible. Administration, to be effective, must result in a balance between staff, service, and money, and thus, any change in any part of either an agency's or a community's nursing program, personnel, or budget necessitates reorganization. For example, what are the implications for a large, established visiting nurse association servicing an entire community, when a new neighborhood health center is established in a housing development with 2000 residents? Does the visiting nurse association continue some of the nursing services for these residents through contractual agreements? If this is the plan, is its nursing staff adequately prepared, or will an in-service education program be necessary? If the neighborhood health center employs its own staff, what about the nursing personnel already employed by the visiting nurse association? Can the agency afford to keep this staff, to expand its program in other directions, and develop other new services, or will it be forced to reduce its staff? How will this affect the cost of a nursing visit? Cost analysis methods have been developed over the years to determine the cost of a nursing visit. This cost unit is used as a basis for both planning and justifying budgets.

Reorganization of an established nursing service may involve development of a different pattern for utilization of staff. A new team plan, for example, may necessitate not only changes in composition of community health nursing staff, with the addition of registered nurses, licensed practical nurses, and perhaps nurses' aides, but also new job descriptions and classification. It may be necessary to develop both an orientation and staff development program. It may also mean employment of a community health nursing specialist as team leader, or the provision of a different kind of supervision to better meet the diverse needs of the members of the nursing team.

Discussion of the administrative implications resulting from change within the nursing system is not included to suggest that the status quo should be maintained. Change is not only desirable but inevitable. Administrative implications, however, must be anticipated. It might be possible, in regard to the example of the neighborhood health center previously mentioned, that a reciprocal arrangement could be worked out between the neighborhood center and the visiting nurse association by which the visiting nurse association might provide some of the staff of the nursing center, thus maintaining some administrative balance within the agency and avoiding duplication of service within the community. The importance of freedom to develop new and better patterns of nursing service and the possible danger of one agency controlling another through such arrangements must always be kept in mind.

Change in the health delivery system will affect and change the administration patterns of community health nursing. For example, in model cities programs nursing aides and lay community coordinators are intimately involved in carrying out part of the nursing program and also in planning it. Other programs, through multidiscipline teams, are making possible a broader than ever approach to health and nursing.

Not only are nursing service and nursing administration changing and affecting each other, but also the structure within which nursing operates, community health, is changing. Society itself is constantly influenced by the needs of an exploding population, spectacular scientific developments resulting in trips to the moon, and the many other urgent and shifting forces of a highly developed technologic society. Within this changing scene new patterns of service and new health workers with different roles and responsibilities will be introduced and old ones abolished. It is inevitable and desirable that community health nursing will change, as it constantly attempts to meet the nursing needs of contemporary society. It is for this reason that the authors have focused on the nursing process, as this will remain essentially constant.

Evaluating the Nursing Plan for the Community

The final step in the process of community health nursing is the evaluation or measurement of the validity of the nursing plan of action which has been developed for the community, in relation to its desired goals. There can be no justification for the existence of any plan or program, particularly one concerned with the health of the community, without assurance of its effectiveness and value. These cannot be just assumed, but must be based on objective and supporting evidence. Evaluation during the planning process and evaluation of the plan of action which has been developed help community health nursing to keep its eyes on the goals, to keep its feet on the ground, and to make decisions along the way with the confidence that comes from knowing that it is headed in the right direction. Evaluation helps to ensure that the decisions which are made are based on objective evidence which can only result from evaluation.

Evaluation has never been more important than it is today. A short supply of personnel, resources, and money, coupled with a multitude of health problems, makes it imperative that new ways be developed to utilize the resources that are available, and to provide evidence of the effectiveness of their utilization. This can be done only through evaluation.

The multiplicity of today's community health problems which confront nursing makes evaluation of the contribution of nursing to their solution extremely important. Community health nursing must constantly seek better ways to evaluate its effectiveness. Nursing programs which do not contribute to the solution of health problems in the community must be discarded or revised, and new ones developed. The health of the population is too important, and the health resources too precious for either ineffective or inefficient nursing programs.

In evaluating community health nursing, progress toward the nursing goals must be the focus, rather than the program of any individual agency within the community. Too often, evidence of progress has been based on annual statistical reports of the numbers and categories of patients served and kinds of services provided rather than on the extent to which the nursing goals for the community have been met. In an attempt to clarify this approach, evaluation will be looked at from two vantage points: first, continuous evaluation during the entire process; and second, evaluation of the plan of action which has resulted.

Throughout the discussion of each step of the process, many evaluative questions have been raised and answers sought. Health problems were determined from the broad health needs of the community and based on a totality of data. Part of this determination involved evaluating health and nursing services against such desirable criteria as comprehensiveness; continuity and coordination; availability, accessibility, and acceptability; and adequacy in terms of resources and facilities. The nursing needs, derived from health problems, were evaluated in relation to the priority of both the health problems and overall nursing needs of the community. Determination of short- and long-range goals was based on careful consideration of many factors, such as whether they were realistic, feasible, and acceptable—both for the community and community health nursing; and what their relationship was to the broader health problems. The goals were stated in clear, measurable, behavioral terms which in turn provided built-in measuring rods for progress toward attainment and effectiveness.

Before the best plan of action was selected, stress was placed on the importance of identifying key leaders and communicators within the community for their sanction and support, and also on the importance of recognizing the contribution of those who because of power, politics, special knowledge, or commitment might make a particular contribution to the success or failure of the plan of action. Other factors considered were timing, community dynamics, and appropriateness. Finally, many evaluative aspects of implementation were explored, such as ways in which change within one community health nursing program affects another, and also the implications of change in regard to the administration of nursing services.

It is evident that evaluation is and must be an inherent part of each step of the process of community health nursing. It provides evidence of progress, guidelines for planning, and a sound basis for decision making. It also guarantees for the consumer safeguards to ensure that the nursing service which he receives will be effective in meeting his nursing needs.

Equally important as evaluation during the planning process is the evaluation of the nursing plan of action which results. This evaluation provides evidence about how well the nursing goals have been met and also whether the goals are important in relation to the overall health problems of the community. For example, the goal in the community that "all adolescent girls pregnant out of wedlock will receive nursing supervision" may well be attained to a considerable extent. This might be accomplished, however, at the expense of other pressing needs within the community, such as the need for nursing care and supervision of patients with chronic disease. Also, was the cost in terms of time, money, effort, or priority of the program too great for the amount of the accomplishment?

Since the goals were stated in terms of observable behavior, they provide yardsticks for objective evidence of the degree to which the desired goals have been attained. For example, if a nursing goal is that "all premature infants in a community will receive nursing supervision in their homes," progress toward this goal can be measured by actually comparing the number of premature babies who receive nursing supervision with the number born who live in a particular community. In addition to evaluating progress toward goals, there are other supporting data that influence success or failure of a program, such as numbers of people who avail themselves of particular nursing services, patterns of utilization, personnel and consumer satisfaction, community involvement and sanction, feasibility in terms of cost, resources, and personnel, and priority in relation to other health needs.

Nursing is part of the overall health care system. Therefore, changes within the health care system are a rough measure of the success or failure of nursing's contribution. For example, reduction of the infant death rate, maternal mortality rate, or disease incidence reflects the contribution of nursing as well as other health professions and other disciplines to the solution of these health problems.

Evaluation of the focus and emphasis of the nursing program within the community in relation to health maintenance, disease prevention, and health promotion, and of the priority accorded to each of these broad areas helps to ensure a well-balanced program. If the major effort of a nursing program is directed toward bedside care, what happens to health promotion and disease prevention? Nursing priorities and programs must always be kept in balance.

Finally, the overall pattern by which community health nursing develops within a community needs to be studied in relationship to the trends and patterns of the broader community—regionalization, comprehensiveness, and finally, a national health plan. Thus, community health nursing must set its sights broadly and determine what and how it can best contribute to the solution of the community's health. It must determine goals by which to make this contribution and strive to measure progress and accomplishment. This can be done through evaluation.

Throughout Part II we have looked critically at each step of the process involved in community health nursing practice with the family as the patient, and again with the community as the patient. Irrespective of where the community health nurse works—in schools, in homes, with groups, industry, public health agencies, ambulatory services, neighborhood health centers, a region, a district, a census tract, and so forth—the process is equally applicable in each situation. Although every situation in which she works will be different and the facts and content will vary, the process which includes collecting data, analyzing the data and identifying the nursing needs, determining the nursing care plan, implementing the care plan, and evaluating the plan will remain essentially the same.

REFERENCES

American Public Health Association. Glossary of evaluative terms in public health. Amer. J. Public Health, 60:1546-1552, August 1970.

Creditor, M. The neighborhood health center: Where does the hospital fit? Amer. J. Public Health, 61:807-813, April 1971.

Ellul, J. The Technological Society. New York, Alfred A. Knopf, 1964.

Freeman, H. E., Levine, S., and Reeder, L. G. Handbook of Medical Sociology. Englewood, N. J., Prentice-Hall, Inc., 1963.

Freeman, R. Community Health Nursing Practice. Philadelphia, W. B. Saunders Company, 1970.

Griffith, E. I. Where do the VNA's go from here? Nurs. Outlook, 16:29-31, March 1968.

Hilleboe, H. E. Public health in the United States in the 1970's. Amer. J. Public Health, 58:1588-1610, September 1968.

Levine, E. Nurse manpower—yesterday, today,and tomorrow. Amer. J. Nurs., 69:290-296, February 1969.

Lewis, C. E. The thermodynamics of regional planning. Amer. J. Public Health, 59:773-777, May 1969.

National League for Nursing. Accreditation of Community Nursing Services. New York, National League for Nursing, 1966, p. 415.

Roberts, D. How effective is public health nursing? Amer. J. Public Health, 52:1077-1083, July 1962.

Robischon, P. Community nursing in a changing climate. Nurs. Outlook, 19:410-413, June 1971.

Sanders, I. T. The Community. New York, The Ronald Press Company, 1958.

Warren, R. L. The Community in America. Chicago, Rand and McNally, 1963.

Wylie, C. M. The definition and measurement of health and disease. Public Health Reports, 85:100-104, February 1970.

PART III

IMPLICATIONS
FOR THE FUTURE

CHAPTER 15
The Road Ahead

The best of times can also be the worst of times. Supersonic planes booming over traffic-clogged highways; tree-lined suburbs and decaying inner cities; zooming salaries and endless welfare lines; exploding knowledge and pervading illiteracy; more and more people for fewer and fewer jobs; democracy and civil rights demonstrations. This is America in the seventies. Dynamism, change, and contrast have always been characteristic of this country. It has from the very beginning been tempered and molded by struggle, strife, and turmoil. Today, however, the tempo of change is accelerating at a geometric rate, with more people, more cars, more demonstrations, and multiplying problems.

The health care delivery system is equally chaotic and on the threshhold of a massive reorganization. One cannot predict just what kind of a system is evolving, but no one will deny that drastic revisions are in process. The current health care system, which is rightfully referred to as a nonsystem, is characterized by specialization, fragmentation, and proliferation, with resulting gaps and duplication; crisis orientation, with lack of long range planning; complexity and automation, with resulting depersonalization. The time has come when the American people will no longer tolerate this kind of care with its escalating costs and inadequate services. Their rising expectations and increasingly insistent demands for more readily available and more effective health care have been to some avail, with discernible organizational patterns gradually coming into focus. No one is clear about exactly what form they will take, but some of the elements or characteristics are predictable at this time, such as:

1. Services will be provided by a multidiscipline team. Many health professionals and consumers will be involved as members of the health team.

2. Services will be comprehensive, with a variety of prepaid group insurance plans, comprehensive neighborhood health centers, and health maintenance organizations.

3. Care outside of the hospital will receive greater emphasis with provisions for services to people wherever they are.

4. Patient care facilities will be increasingly automated and complex due to the knowledge explosion and scientific and technologic developments.

5. Health care will be organized in such a way that entrance into it and orderly progression within it will be facilitated.

6. A national health insurance plan will become a reality, although its form and structure is unclear at present. Undoubtedly, health will finally become a public utility.

The period of transition between the present chaotic nonsystem and the emerging system of health care will be painful and exciting. Community health nursing, with all other professional persons, is part of this scene. It is also experiencing rapid change, with old patterns, methods, and long traditions being shattered and new patterns and developments as yet not stabilized. This is an era in which nothing will remain static for any length of time, and decisions made today may not be valid tomorrow. The future of community health nursing in this changing milieu is uncertain. How it responds will either make it a potent force in shaping the health care system of the future or consign it to oblivion.

No professional group shapes its own destiny, but it can take advantage of the available opportunities to determine the directions in which it should go. The evolution of community health nursing is dotted with periods of crisis and uncertainty. It has responded at some times by assuming leadership and forging ahead; and at others by marking time and keeping the status quo. It is risky to predict what the future holds for community health nursing. However, we believe it has the elements and the potential for making a significant contribution to society if it utilizes its wisdom, energy, and creativity to harness these assets for maximum effectiveness.

Community health nursing has a vast storehouse of knowledge about health problems of families and an awareness gained from long experience about their hopes and aspirations. From the beginning its locus of operation has been in the community, and its main focus has been the relationship of the health of the family to the health of the community. Community health nursing in general, however, has not taken the initiative in sharing its knowledge and concerns with others, or in assuming leadership in mobilizing appropriate people and resources for social action. By developing increased astuteness and knowledge about the politics of power, the sources of money, and the legislative channels of government, it could become a potent force in bringing about needed changes in community health. Community health nursing encompasses the largest group of prepared community health workers and has the ability and experience to assume a leadership role and play a social activist role in relation to health.

In the decade ahead the demands by the people for determining the kinds of health services they desire, and for working in partnership with professionals in planning for these services, will move into high gear. The requirement of much of the federal legislation for maximum feasible participation of the consumers in planning health programs will further their participation. Community health nursing has a longer tradition than any other group in working in partnership with citizens in planning and implementing community health nursing programs. It has great opportunities to translate this knowledge to other professional groups who are struggling to become partners with consumers and at the same time retain their own professional identities.

The rapid development and expansion of health services, coupled with the proliferation of specialists of all kinds, has resulted in confusion, and in some instances veritable chaos, within the community. It is, in the last analysis, the patient who is caught in trying to find his way into or through this tortuous network. Patients and families desperately need someone to help them find where to turn, to support them during crises, to coordinate the multiplicity of services and resources, to mobilize the resources, and to speak in their behalf. Community health nurses because of their long experience in collaborating with others in the community and in utilizing community resources, plus their acceptance as helping persons by people in their own homes, can readily assume the coordinative and caring responsibility for which families are pleading, and can become their advocate on health matters.

One of the results of the knowledge explosion is, and will continue to be, an even greater increase in specialization of health workers, with each concentrating on one aspect of health in the individual or the community. Specialism will also invade community health nursing, and its expertise will be built on the concepts of the family and the community as the patient. Thus, the community health nurse's practice will be geared to a broad generalist approach, and she might well be defined as a "generalized specialist." By building upon the skills she already has and developing further expertise, the community health nurse can help families integrate the services they are receiving. The impression that in these days one goes to one physician or health facility for a left foot, and to another for a right ear, is not too far from the truth. One might ask who really is concerned about the whole patient—much less the whole family. The fragmentation which has resulted from specialization is frightening and potentially hazardous. Never was the need for a generalist more pressing—and the community health nurse can fill that need.

As we look ahead at the shape of things to come and consider the possible directions and potential contribution of community health nursing within this evolving health system, we believe that community health nursing will become the professional group to provide primary health care to families. It has always assumed part of this responsibility and has considerable knowledge and experience as a basis for further development of this role. Community health nursing is already carrying out many of the functions once thought to be those of the general practitioner. Some of these are:

1. It has long assessed the health needs of individuals within the family, and of the family as a whole.
2. It has made judgments about whether medical care is needed, what kind, and where it is to be obtained.
3. It has coordinated various health services and interpreted medical orders.

4. It has helped to improve health practices of the family and has pre-scribed time-tested remedies.

5. It has recognized the value of cultural and ethnic practices and has exploited these to the advantage of the families.

6. It has intervened and supported families during periods of stress and crisis.

These and many other long-standing activities of community health nursing need to be legitimatized. However, in order to become effective as family health nurse practitioners in the evolving health care system, community health nursing will need additional know-ledge and tools. Some of these are:

1. To further explore and clarify the independent functions of the nurse, as well as her dependent and interdependent functions.

2. To add to its armamentarium some tools, previously considered the prerogative of the physician, such as physical assessment of indivi-duals. There is nothing magical about using instruments such as the stethoscope or the otoscope, and there is no reason why these should not be used by the community health nurse.

3. To become more skillful in making judgements about the medical care and treatment a family needs and in prescribing some of the diagnostic tests basic to determining the appropriate point of entry into the medical care system.

4. To develop greater depth of knowledge of growth and development of individuals, and of the common ailments of various age groups.

With this and other appropriate knowledge community health nursing can more effectively develop its role as family health nurse practitioners. These added responsibilities are all logical extensions of the nursing role.

The role of the community health nurse as the family health nurse practitioner is only one of the new roles she will assume in the evolving health care system. She will work as a full-fledged member of a multidiscipline team in meeting the health needs of people. She also will be working with others in the community in identifying health problems and in planning community health programs.

In order for the emerging health care system to be effective, the education of health workers will undergo a metamorphosis. No longer will each discipline educate its practitioners in isolation with-out regard to the changing roles and responsibilities of other profes-sionals. A common core of knowledge necessary for every health worker will be identified, and core courses and curricula plans will be developed. This will provide an opportunity for student health personnel to be educated together and to understand the contributions of each other. By having a common core of knowledge, it will also be possible for students to change their career choices without being penalized by having to start their education all over again.

With a core curriculum it will be even more important for each discipline to identify its contribution to health care and to demonstrate its value. This is as equally true of nursing and community health nursing as of all other disciplines. If nursing is to become a full-fledged partner of the health team, its members must have equal education preparation. In this technologic era with its high premium on education, an apprentice type preparation for professional practice will no longer suffice. Nursing must move into the mainstream of higher education in order to realize its full potential in the seventies.

The decade ahead will be a period of experimentation with various educational patterns. Many of the experiments, such as short-term programs for the expanded role of the nurse, will continue to develop outside of educational institutions in order to meet the specific needs of special age groups or disease categories. Oftentimes through these kinds of experiments, new pathways can be opened up for significant developments of the profession. However, they must be evaluated very carefully, and those aspects which further the development of nursing as a profession should be retained and included as part of the educational preparation of all nurses. Those aspects which do not enhance the profession should be abolished.

The National Commission for the Study of Nursing and Nursing Education[1] has recommended the development of two differing career patterns for nursing practice. One is termed *episodic*, and is defined as nursing practice that is essentially curative and restorative, treating ailments that are acute and chronic in nature, and provided in hospitals or other patient care facilities. The other is termed *distributive*, and is defined as nursing practice essentially geared to health maintenance and disease prevention which is continuous in nature, seldom acute, and takes place in the community or emergent institutional settings. The implications of this report for nursing education, and of the report of the Carnegie Commission on Higher Education in relation to medical and dental education will have to be scrutinized very critically in the movement toward core curricula for all health students.

[1] National Commission for the Study of Nursing and Nursing Education. *An Abstract for Action*. New York, McGraw-Hill Book Company, 1970, p. 92.

Due to a variety of factors, such as age shifts in the population and the average age of teachers who are now employed, there will be fewer job opportunities for teachers now and in the next decade. Consequently, there will be an abundance of young people and college graduates, both male and female, who may be attracted into the health field. Some of these will select nursing as a career. This will necessitate expanding baccalaureate programs, as well as developing postbaccalaureate nursing programs for the college graduate. Undoubtedly, the impact of larger numbers of men in nursing, and of nursing on men, will be major, as has happened in other predominantly female occupations when men became an inherent part.

Specialization and advanced educational programs will expand, and graduate education will become accepted increasingly as the basis for expertise in nursing practice. The continuous flow of new knowledge, generated by science, technology, and research, will necessitate constant reevaluation of graduate content for its relevance to expert practice. Mechanisms should also be set up for a continuous and orderly movement of appropriate content to flow into baccalaureate nursing programs.

We believe that preparation of the family health nurse practitioner should and will become an inherent part of the preparation of the community health nursing specialist. It is this nurse, with graduate preparation in community health nursing, who will become the skilled family nurse practitioner. She is the person who will be collaborating with multidiscipline teams in comprehensive health centers. She will also have a peer relationship with other clinical nursing specialists—and will use her expertise to coordinate these services for the family as a whole. She is the person who must take leadership in evolving and demonstrating the contribution of community health nursing in solving the health problems of families and communities.

There is an urgent need for research in nursing in relation to the clinical practice, the education of nurses, and the nursing care delivery system. The need for this is not new but has been pointed out repeatedly by many during the past several years. The need to develop the science of nursing and to be able to better determine what we do that makes a difference, and how we might discover other and better ways to care for patients is urgent. Whatever the reasons may be for the paucity of clinical research to date, the road ahead looks more promising. Renewed interest in and concern for clinical practice,

with accompanying expansion of specialized graduate nursing programs, has resulted in a growing reservoir of well-prepared and highly
motivated nurses. These specialists bring new focus and commitment
as well as knowledge and skill to their particular fields of interest,
and community health nursing specialists are part of this group.

Because the community health nurse specialist—hopefully the
family health nurse practitioner of the future—is closely involved in
caring for the patient and his family, she is in a strategic position to
identify nursing problems that need to be studied. In order to
improve practice, she must identify and document what she is doing,
develop and test hypotheses, and contribute to theories for nursing
practice. Many of the nursing problems in the home seem to be
different from those in the hospital, but are they? How is effectiveness of nursing intervention measured? What nursing decisions are
made by the nurse, and what is the effect on the family? Are the
community patterns for providing nursing care effective? How can
this be measured? These are only a few examples of the kinds of
questions which need to be raised and for which answers should be
sought. When there are specialists in community health nursing, it is
much more likely that problems in practice will be identified, and
research initiated.

Equally important as clinical research is research regarding new
curricula patterns. The system of nursing education, similar to the
health system, is characterized by confusion and fragmentation.
What is the best way to prepare nurses for a rapidly changing health
care system? How can one devise a nursing education program that
will allow for orderly entrance and progression of those with varying
educational levels and backgrounds? How can educational programs
continuously integrate new and expanding knowledge? How can they
be more relevant to the needs of a changing, dynamic society? These
and many other pertinent questions must be raised and answers
sought.

No one will deny that community health nursing has a great deal
of hard work ahead—to improve its practice, its system of delivering
care, and its education. It has, however, already come a long way and
through other anxious periods of history. Community health nursing
will continue to evolve and change. It will continue to be influenced
by an interplay of societal forces and to be a force in itself. It is

because of this dynamism of the world in which we live that in this book we have focused on the process of community health nursing— as this process will remain essentially unchanged in a changing world. There are exciting times ahead. Community health nursing has the potential to make a contribution to the health of the people. We believe it also has the wisdom, energy, and creativity.

REFERENCES

Editorial. Empirical research in nursing. Nurs. Res., 20:99, March-April 1971.
—— Research in nursing—a critical need. Nurs. Res., 20:195, May-June 1971.
Carnegie Commission of Higher Education. Higher Education and the Nation's Health. New York, McGraw-Hill Book Company, 1970.
Drucker, P. F. The surprising seventies. Harpers, 243:35-39, July 1971.
National Commission for the Study of Nursing and Nursing Education. An Abstract for Action. New York, McGraw-Hill Book Company, 1970.

Family Data Collection

Name of family_____

Address_____

I. Family Characteristics

   A. Persons living in the household

Name	Date of Birth	Sex	Race	Relation to Head of House	Occupation

   B. Members of family not living in household

C. Roles of members—what are assigned household tasks?

Adults

Children

D. Relationships of members—how do they get along?

Husband-wife

Father-children

Mother-children

Children-children

E. Decision making—who makes them? How?

Major decisions

Minor decisions

F. Sleeping arrangements

Which family members sleep together?

Which family members sleep alone?

What type of bed does each have?

What are the usual hours of sleep?   Bedtime   Arise   Rest periods

Adults

Children

G. Eating patterns

Observation about kitchen and mealtimes

Observations of family members for nutritional status

24-hour family-food intake beginning with previous day's breakfast

Breakfast

Lunch

Dinner

Snacks

H. Leisure—what are the usual activities?

Adults

Children

II. Socioeconomic and Cultural Factors

A. Educational level—what is the highest school grade completed?

Adults

Children

B. Ethnic group background

C. Religious affiliation

D. Occupation of working members

E. Income

Family income $_____(week, month, year)

Source—Salary $_____ Savings $ _____ Investments $_____
   Pensions $_____ Social Security $_____Veterans $_____
   AFDC $_____Welfare $_____
   Other $ _____

Contributions of working members
Member_____Amount $_____(week, month, year)

Are expenses greater or less than income?
greater   less   equal

Who plans how the money is spent?

F. Social relations—who do the family members interact with outside of the immediate family, and what community activities do they participate in?

Extended family_____
Neighbors_____
Friends_____
Church_____
Clubs_____
Community activities (list) _____
_____
Other_____

G. Value system

Observations of nurse

Home _____
Furniture_____
Neighborhood _____
Other _____

Comments by mother or other family members

III. Environmental Factors

A. Housing

Type_____Own_____Rent_____
Number of rooms_____ Furniture adequate_____inadequate_____
Type of refrigeration for food_____
Toilet facilities—inside_____outside_____
Water supply—municipal_____well_____other_____
Flies—yes_____ no_____
Rodents—yes_____ no_____
Accident hazards (list)

B. Neighborhood

Residential_____ industrial_____ rural_____
urban _____ ghetto _____ suburban _____ other_____

Type of dwellings

Condition of dwellings

Accessibility of play areas—Yes   No

Accessibility of health facilities—Yes   No
(list)

Accessibility of churches—Yes   No

Accessibility of schools—Yes   No

C. Transportation

Public transportation—Yes   No
            Adequate   Yes   No
Other

IV. Health and Medical History

A. Present illnesses of each member

B. Is any family member taking any medication—Yes   No
        If "yes", name of drug, how often taken, and by whom?

C. History of past significant illnesses and accidents of each member

D. Immunization status of each member

E. How is medical care financed?

Medical insurance_____   Medicare_____
Hospital insurance_____   Medicaid_____
Own finances_____   Other_____

F. What is the state of dental health of each member?

G. What is the knowledge and attitude of the family about health?

H. What does the family perceive as its health problems?

I. What does the nurse perceive as the family health problems?

J. What has been the previous experience of the family with the community health nurse? What did she do?

K. What does the family think is the reason for present visit by the nurse?

L. What are the nursing needs as seen by the family?

M. What is the family's expectation of the community health nurse?

N. How has the family managed in previous situations of illness or crisis?

Own resources _____
Extended family_____
Other relatives _____
Friends_____
Neighbors _____
Significant others_____
Other _____

O. How will family manage between visits of community health nurse?

V. Summary

A. What are the family health problems?

B. To which of the family health problems <u>can</u> nursing make a contribution?

C. To which of the family health problems <u>should</u> nursing make a contribution? Why?

D. Which of the family health problems should nursing <u>leave alone</u>? Why?

E. What are the family nursing needs that you will give first priority? Second priority? Third priority? And so forth.

APPENDIX B
Community Nursing Survey Guide

Community_____Date of Survey_____

I. The Community

   A. Description: Include general identifying data, i.e., location, topography, climate, urban, rural, etc.

   B. Boundaries: Specific boundaries surrounding study area

   C. Area in square miles

   D. Population per square mile

E. Mobility of population

F. Type of government—community legislative programs

G. History: Include significant changes such as urban development, major highway construction, regionalization, shifts in industry

H. Community changes anticipated

II. Population Characteristics

A. Population and age distribution

	Community				State		National	
Age Group	Current Population 19____	Percent	Population 10 years ago	Percent	Population	Percent	Population	Percent
0-5								
5-14								
15-24								
25-34								
35-44								
45-54								
55-64								
65-74								
75+								

B. Sex and race distribution—19_____

		Community		State		National	
Race	Sex	Number	Percent	Number	Percent	Number	Percent
Nonwhite	Female						
	Male						
White	Female						
	Male						
Total							

C. Ethnic group composition—19_____

	Community		State		National	
Race	Number	Percent	Number	Percent	Number	Percent

D. Religious distribution—19_____

	Community		State		National	
Religion	Number	Percent	Number	Percent	Number	Percent
Catholic						
Protestant						
Jewish						
Other						

E. Educational levels (persons 25+) 19_____

Percent of Population

Education	Percent	Percent	Percent
No Schooling			
1-4 Years			
5-8 Years			
Attended High School			
Graduate from High School			
Attended College			
Median Years of Education			

F. Socioeconomic characteristics

1. Income of families—19_____

Percent of families

Income	Community Percent	State Percent	Federal Percent
Under $3,000			
$3,000–5,999			
$6,000–9,999			
$10,000 +			
Median Income			

2. Leading industries

Name	Address	No. Employed
_____	_____	_____
_____	_____	_____
_____	_____	_____

3. Occupations (list categories)

_____ _____

_____ _____

_____ _____

4. Estimated level of unemployment

Community_____ State_____ National _____

III. Environmental Factors

A. General description of environment

B. Housing

1. Condition of housing

Type of Dwelling	Good		Fair		Poor	
	No.	Percent	No.	Percent	No.	Percent

2. Ownership and rental status

Percent

Units owned _____
Units rented _____

C. Sanitation

1. Water supply, sewage, trash, and garbage

   Source of Water Supply   Public _____ Private _____
   Sewage Disposal   Public _____ Private _____
   Trash and Garbage   Public _____ Private _____

D. Protection

1. Fire protection (describe) _____

2. Police protection (describe) _____

3. Civil defense (describe) _____

4. Safety (describe significant safety programs or hazards)

   _____

   _____

E. Transportation

   Describe transportation systems: bus, suburban train, air,
                                          private automobile, other

F. Other significant environmental factors

IV. Communication Resources

A. News media
   newspapers

Name	Publication Schedule	Circulation
_____	_____	_____
_____	_____	_____
_____	_____	_____

B. Radio stations (local)

C. Television

D. Key community leaders (list and identify)

E. Other

V. Health Information

A. Vital statistics 19_____

	Community		State		National	
	Number	Rate	Number	Rate	Number	Rate
Live births						
Neonatal deaths						
Infant deaths						
Maternal deaths						
Deaths						

B. Disease incidence and prevalence 19_____

Disease	Community				State				National			
	Number		Rate		Number		Rate		Number		Rate	
	I	P	I	P	I	P	I	P	I	P	I	P
Cardiovascular												
Cancer												
Diabetes												
Other significant												

C. Leading causes of death*

	Community		State	National
Cause of Death	Number	Rate	Rate	Rate
1.				
2.				
3.				
4.				
5.				
6.				
7.				
8.				
9.				
10.				

VI. Health Facilities and Resources

A. Hospitals

Name

1) Ownership
2) Accreditation, type
3) Average hospitalization

Type Service

medical _____   psychiatric _____
surgical _____   communicable
maternity_____   disease _____
pediatric _____   intensive care _____
rehabilitation _____   chronic disease _____

*Include other information and/or statistics significant for your community and compare with state and national figures.

B. Nursing homes

Name

Ownership _____
Accreditation _____
Certification _____
Bed capacity _____
Services _____
Other_____

C. Ambulatory Services

Name of hospital or clinic

Emergency_____   Drug Addiction_____
Maternity_____   Alcoholism_____
Pediatric_____   Psychiatric_____
Family Planning_____ Dental_____
Medical_____   Eye_____
Surgical_____   Other_____
Orthopedic_____

D. Other health care resources

   1. Occupational health services

   2. School health services

   3. Health departments

   4. Voluntary health agencies

   5. Comprehensive health centers (model cities, neighborhood centers, Maternal & Infant, Children & Youth, etc.)

   6. Prepaid group health plans

   7. Other

E. Health-related planning groups (i.e., Council of Health and Social Agencies, Health Council, etc.)

Identify and briefly describe purpose, people served, personnel of these resources, and services extended to the community.

F. Health personnel

Personnel	No. Living in Community	No. Active
Physician		
Dentist		
Registered Nurse		
Licensed Practical Nurse		
Physical Therapist		
Sanitary Engineers		
Social Workers		
Occupational Therapists		
Significant Others		

VII. Community Health Nursing Services

A. Identifying data

1. Name of agency
2. Purpose of agency

3. Legal authority
4. Certified Home Health Agency   Yes   No
   Date of certification
5. Accredited (APHA-NLN)   Yes   No
   Date accredited
6. Organization: (describe and/or include Table of Organization)

7. Administration
   (1) Board of Directors
       a. Number of board members Total   M   F
       b. Community groups or interests represented (list)

    c. Maximum number of consecutive terms possible for a board member
    d. Frequency of general board meetings

    e. Regular attendance at board meetings by Nursing Director
       Yes   No
    f. Committees of the board (list)

(2) Nursing Director
    a. Job description

    b. Lines of authority

B. Finances
  1. Income
      Capital funds and endowment
      Tax funds (list sources)

      Earnings
        Fees from patients _____
        Insurance _____
        Medicare _____
        Medicaid _____
        Welfare _____
        Other (list) _____

      All other income (grants, refunds, etc.)

      Total Income

2. Expenditures
   Salaries
   　　Director _____
   　　Supervisor _____
   　　Assistant Supervisor _____
   　　Consultants
   　　　　Nursing _____
   　　　　Nonnursing _____
   　　Clinical Nurse Specialist _____
   　　Community Health Nurse _____
   　　Registered Nurse _____
   　　Licensed Practical Nurse _____
   　　Home Health Aide _____
   　　Neighborhood Aide _____
   　　Clerical _____
   　　Other _____

   In-service Education _____
   Transportation _____
   Nursing Supplies and Equipment _____
   Rent and Related Expenses _____
   Office Expenses (records, telephone, etc.) _____
   All other general expenses (specify) _____

   Total Expenses _____

3. Method used to determine cost per unit

   Date
   Cost per visit
   Charge for visit　　　　　　　　　　Date established

C. Personnel
  1. Professional nursing personnel

	No.	Educ. Prep.	Total Exper- ience CHN	Length of Experience with the Agency	Part-Time	Full-Time
Executive Director						
Supervisor						
Assistant Supervisor						
Clinical Nurse Specialist						
Nurse Consultant						
Staff Community Health Nurses						
Registered Nurses						

  2. Other professional personnel

	No.	Educ. Prep.	No. of Years With Agency	Full-Time	Part-Time
Physician					
Physical Therapist					
Occupational Therapist					
Social Worker					
Statistician					
Nutritionist					
Sanitarian					
Health Educator					

3. Other personnel*

	No.	No. of Years With Agency	Full-Time	Part-Time
Licensed Practical Nurse				
Home Health Aide				
Neighborhood Aide				
Clerical Staff				
Other (list)				

4. Volunteers

No. of hours of assistance available last year—19_____
Activities carried by volunteers (list)

5. Utilization of personnel

a. Team plan (describe)

1) Composition of team
2) Qualifications and responsibilities of members

b. Rationale for nursing responsibilities

1) Districts
2) Type of care
3) Preparation of staff

c. Job descriptions

D. Services

1. Total cases   Visits   in 19_____

*Indicate type of responsibilities.

2. Care of the Sick

Classification of Illness	Cases	Visits	Percentage of Total Visits
Cancer			
Heart Disease			
Diabetes			
Others (list)			
Tuberculosis			
Venereal Disease			
Other Communicable Diseases (list)			

3. Health guidance

Classification	Cases	Visits	Percentage of Total Visits
Maternity Antepartal			
Postpartal			
Infant Premature			
Neonatal other than Premature			
Other—1 Year			
Preschool			
School			
Adult			
Adult 65+			

4. Clinic service

Type of Clinic	No. Sessions per Month	Attendance per Session	Total Monthly Attendance	Nurses per Session	Other Personnel per Session

5. School health service

Type of School	No. of Schools	Pupil Enrollment	No. of Teachers
Nursery			
Elementary			
Secondary			
Special Ed.			
Day Care Centers			
Head Start			
Total			

6. Comprehensive Health, Neighborhood Health, or Model Cities (describe nursing program)

7. Other services

Identify and describe other nursing services and/or programs involving Community Health Nursing, such as those relating to Occupational Health, Family Planning, Drug Addiction, Alcoholism, Community Mental Health, Parent Teaching, or other.

E. Referrals and contracts

1. Sources of referral for community health nursing

Hospitals (including OPD)
Home Care Programs
Prepaid Group Plans
Other Agencies
Family or Patient
Friend
Community Health Nurse
Other (indicate)

2. System for referral between community health nursing services within the community (describe)

3. Contractual agreements with other community agencies for community health nursing services (identify and describe)

Index

Accidents, 228, 231
Accreditation
    of community services, 95, 113, 216
    of educational programs, 82-83, 93
Action, nursing, 176 ff., 236 ff., 251 ff.
    alternatives, 247 ff.
    change and, 259-60
    for community, 236 ff., 251 ff.
    coordination of, 185-87, 259
    evaluation of, 188 ff., 261 ff.
    for family, 172-74, 176 ff.
    least preparation for, 180-81
    reorganization of existing services and,
        260
    social, 237
    timing for, 244
    unanticipated problems and, 252-53
Activities of family, 135-36
    assisting and complementing of, 173
    community, 140, 141
Administrative patterns, 216, 259, 260
Adolescent pregnant girls, 258

Age
    characteristics of community, 209, 225
    family and, 133
    median, stages of life and, 74
Age of Reform, 37
Agencies
    administration of, 216, 259, 260
    certification of, 215-16
    changes in, 242, 259, 260
    data on, 218, 232-33
    existing, 215 ff.
    extension of services, 255, 258
    funds, 217, 242-43
    implementation of plan and, 254-55
    job description of director, 217
    mobilization of resources and, 256-57
    official, 254-55
    personnel, 217-18
    policies, 123-24, 127
    referrals and, 249-50, 259
    voluntary. See Voluntary health
        agencies.

Air travel, 31, 65
Alexander, John, 196
Allen, F. L., 40
Alternatives in plan of action, 247 ff.
American Association of Junior Colleges, 82
American Nurses' Association
    definition of public health nurse, 93-94
    economic security program, 79
    examinations for licensure, 84
    founding, 43
    reorganization and, 82
    higher education and, 85-86, 88, 98
    World War II and, 80
American Public Health Association, 55, 95
    accreditation of community services,
        216
American Red Cross, 45
American Society of Superintendents of
        Training Schools for Nurses, 17,
        44, 52
Analysis of data
    for community, 220 ff.
    for family, 146 ff.
"Angel of mercy" image, 97
Apprentice type of education, 16
Armed forces, 74
    Nurse Corps, 80
    recruitment in World War II, 44
Assembly line, 30
Associate degree programs, 84, 87, 112
Association of Collegiate Schools of
        Nursing, 47, 82
Atom bomb, 66
Automobile, 30-31, 64
Autonomous functions, 125
Autonomous nuclear family, 120-21
    dependency of, 168, 173
Availability of resources, 179-80, 221,
        233, 234
Avalon Foundation, 88

Baccalaureate programs, 84, 90, 93, 112
Base-line data
    on community, 232-33, 253
    on family, 130-31, 149, 154, 162-63,
        177-78
Beard, Mary, 45
Behavior
    observable, evaluation of, 263
    value system and, 139-40
Bell, D., 69
Bellevue Hospital, 15
Bergman, R. L., 173
Birth rate, 213
Black university students, 73
Blue Cross, 91
Boards of education, 127
Bolton, Frances Payne, 46

Boston, district nursing development and,
        19, 20, 52
Boundaries, community, 207
Brewster, Mary, 21
British immigrants, 33
Brown Report, 81-82
Budget
    agency, 217
    family, 168

Cadet Nurse Corps, 80
Care. See also Health care system; Plan,
        nursing care.
    as focus of nursing, 86
    home programs, 91, 179, 255
    by students, 79
Career patterns, future of, 274
Carnegie, Andrew, 11
Carnegie Commission on Higher Education,
        274
Carnegie Foundation, 39
Carson, Rachael, 67
Causes of death, 230-31
Census Bureau, 49, 213
Census, first, of public health nurses, 54-55
Census tracts, 207-208, 230
Central registry, 259
Central schools of nursing, 81
Certified home health agency, 215-16
Change
    activating plan and, 259-60
    community and, 197, 200, 202-203,
        252, 259-60
    consumers and, 203
    facilities and, 214
    family and, 181-83
    goals and, public health, 201
    health delivery system and, 260-61
    implementation of plan and, 252
Charitable work. See also Voluntary health
        agencies.
    settlements and, 20 ff., 38
Charity
    beginnings of, 11
    community chests, 39, 76
Child health program, 241
Children, nuclear family and, 120
Children's Bureau, 38
Cities
    automobile and, 64
    ghetto areas of, 106, 210
    model, 107, 261
    poverty and, 70
    schools of, 71
    settlements in, 20 ff., 38
    suburbanization and, 70, 106
    visiting nurse services in, 51
Citizen groups, 24-25, 50, 59-60

Civil rights movement, 71, 73, 77
Civil Service Commissions, 90
Civil War aftermath, 3 ff.
Clayton Act (1914), 32
Cleveland, 39, 52
Clinical practice
    priority of, 86, 111
    research, future of, 275-76
Collaboration
    for community, 113, 114, 219, 257
    for family, 162, 177, 183-84
Collection of people, community as, 195
College Settlement, 22
Colleges and universities
    community, 82
    curricula, 34-35, 71, 79, 274, 276
    diploma programs, 84, 87, 112
    doctoral programs, 87, 88, 97, 112
    enrollment, 72
    federal aid to, 72, 73, 112
    financial plight of, 108
    first Department of Nursing, 52
    G.I. Bill and, 72, 81
    graduate programs, 112. See also Gradu-
        ate programs.
    junior, 34, 71
    master's programs, 84, 87, 88, 112
    in 1970s, 112
    nursing programs, 42-43, 47, 84-86
    preparation for, 71
    recruitment, 43
    student unrest, 73, 78
    visiting nurse associations and, 52
    women's development of, 12-13, 35-36
Committee on the Grading of Nursing
        Schools, 47
Committee on Nursing of the Council of
        National Defense, 44
Committee on Social Trends, 31
Committee for the Study of Nursing Edu-
        cation, 46
Committee on University Schools, 47
Communicable disease, 49
Communications, 212-13, 227, 229, 257
    key people, 212, 229, 263
Community, 193 ff.
    accreditation of services, 95, 113, 216
    age characteristics, 209, 225
    agencies, 243-44
    ascertaining resources of, 254-56
    availability of services, 179-80, 183-84,
        221, 233, 234
    base-line data, 232-33, 253
    boundaries, 207
    census tracts, 207-208, 230
    chest, 76
        first, 39
    collaboration and coordination in, 113,
        114, 185-87, 257, 259

Community (cont.)
    as collection of people, 195
    colleges, 82
    communication channels, 212-13, 227,
        229, 257, 263
    comprehensive care, 113, 231, 241
    data gathering, 196, 205 ff. See also
        Data, community.
    definition of, 194-95
    duplication of responsibilities in, 94
    dynamics of change, 197, 200, 202-203,
        252, 259-60
    economic factors, 53, 223, 226
    educational level, 226
    environmental factors, 210-12, 226 ff.
    equilibrium, 208
    evaluation of plan for, 261 ff.
    existing services in, 215 ff., 251
        expansion of, 258
        reorganization of, 260
    facilities. See Facilities, community.
    family relationship to, 140, 141, 169-
        71, 180
    federal government and, 95, 208, 223
    formal organizations, 197
    functions, 197
    goals for, 240 ff., 262-63
    government of, 208, 223
    health departments, 92, 254-55
    health and illness patterns, 213, 230 ff.
    health nurse, 114
        actions, evaluation of, 188 ff., 261 ff.
        areas of knowledge, 118
        basic assumptions about, 115-16,
            160-61
        competence, 186
        contacts, 174, 180, 184
        continuing development of, 187
        definition of, 114
        focus of, 162, 264, 271
        functions of, 125, 173, 272-73
        future for, 269 ff.
        leadership, 128
        long-standing practices and, 124
        preparation and utilization of, 126-
            28
        responsibilities of, 115
        specialists, 185
    health services, criteria for, 221-22
    history, 208, 223-24
    housing, 210-11, 227
    implementation of plan for, 251 ff.
    income and, 226
    informal organizations, 197
    institutions, family and, 140, 141
    location, 222
    mobility in, 223
    mobilization of resources, 256-57
    nursing needs, identification of, 220 ff.

organized effort of, 202
physical change, 202
as place, 194
planning for, 236 ff.
politics, 243
population characteristics, 208, 209,
    224-26
power, 243
preplanning for, 199, 239-40
profile, 207
protective programs, 202
protective services, 211, 228
public health movement and, 51, 94
resources. See Facilities, community;
    Resources, community.
sex characteristics, 209
size, 208, 222
as social system, 194-95
"of solution," 95, 142, 244, 258
transportation, 212, 228-29
vital statistics, 213, 230
waste disposal, 211, 228
water supply, 211, 228
Comprehensive health care, 95, 221, 231
    centers, 113
    collaboration and, 177
    decision-making and, 199-200
    need for, 86
    planning and, 199-200, 241
Comprehensive Health Planning Act, 199
Conceptual frameworks for nursing, 146-47,
    221
Consultation services, 89
Consumerism, 110, 161, 203
Contacts, nursing, 174, 180, 184
Continuing professional development, 187
Continuous health care, 221
Contractual agreements, 259
Coordinating Council, 82
Coordination of health services, 219, 221,
    257, 259
    for family, 185-87
Core curriculum, 274
Cost study methods, 55, 217
Council of National Defense, 44, 45
Council of State Boards, 84
Counseling, 258
Crandall, Ella Phillips, 44, 45
Cultural factors of family, 137-38, 179
Curative vs. preventive services, 214
Curricula, 34-35, 71, 79, 274, 276

Daily activities of family, 135
Data
    community, 196, 205 ff.
        about people, 209-10
        analysis, 220 ff.

Data (cont.)
    base-line, 232-33, 253
    communications, 212-13, 227, 229,
        257, 263
    environmental, 210-12, 226 ff.
    facilities and resources, 214 ff.
    health information, 213, 230 ff.
    population characteristics, 208, 209,
        224-26
    family, 130 ff.
        analysis, 146 ff.
        base-line, 130-31, 149, 154, 162-63,
            177-78
        demographic, 132, 153
        environmental, 140-42, 153
        health and medical history, 142-44
        nursing needs and, 146 ff.
        organization of, 148
        relationship of items to each other,
            154-55
        socioeconomic and cultural, 137 ff.
DDT, 67
Death
    causes of, 230-31
    rate, 213, 230
Death Registration Area, 49, 213
Debts, family, 137-38
DeCarlo, C. R., 187
Decision-making
    community, 239
    family, 134-135, 149-50, 172
        care plan and, 160-61
        comprehensive care and, 199-200
        implementation of plan and, 178-80
Defensive position of public health nurse,
    93
Demographic data, 132, 153
Department of Nursing and Health, first
    university, 52
Dependency of family, 168, 173
Depression, 40-41, 48, 55, 57
Development of nursing plan
    for community, 236 ff.
    for family, 159 ff.
Developmental aspect of nursing, 152
Developmental stage of family, 132, 147
Diabetes, 172-73
Diagnosis, nursing, definition of, 152
Dietary patterns, 135-36, 171
Dimock, Susan, 15
Diploma programs, 84, 87, 112
Directors, qualifications for, 55, 217
Disease prevention, 169-71, 214
Distribution of goods, 67
Distributive career patterns, 274
District nursing
    development of, 18 ff.
    diversification of activities, 52

first associations, 19
number of organizations in 1900, 22
public health movement and, 50-51
voluntary movement in, 50
Division of Nurse Education (USPHS), 80
Doctoral programs, 87, 88, 97, 112
Drug addiction, 235
Dulles, F., 9, 66
Duplication of resources, 94, 177, 214
Duvall, E., 132, 133

Eating patterns, 135-36, 171
Economics
    community, 53
    depression, 40-41
    family, 137-38, 150, 167, 168
    individual related to community, 53
    monopolies and trusts, 31-32
    production of goods, 66
    security program of ANA, 79
    technology and, 68
    women and, 75
Education
    accreditation of programs, 82-83
    apprentice type, 16
    baccalaureate programs, 84, 90, 93, 112
    Civil War, 4, 6
    community level of, 226
    continuing programs, 187
    costs of, 73
    diploma programs, 84, 87, 112
    doctoral programs, 87, 88, 97, 112
    evaluation of programs, 46-47, 53, 79,
        82-83
    family, 150
    federal funds, 90
    first funds for nursing, 52
    first graduate school, 13
    free public, 12
    future for, 273-74, 276
    higher. See Colleges and universities;
        Graduate programs.
    historical background
        1865 to 1900, 11-13
        1900 to New Deal, 34-36, 46-47, 57
        New Deal to Johnson era, 70 ff.
        1970s, 107-108, 111-12
    individualism and, 13
    legislation, 42
    master's programs, 84, 87, 88, 112
    medical, early, 16
    philanthropy and, 13
    postgraduate programs, 47-48, 53, 88
    practical nurse programs, 84
    priorities in, 112-13
    professionalism and, 84
    qualifications for public health nurse, 55

research, 274, 276
separate but equal, 71
social consciousness and, 76
standards, development of, 52-53, 58, 59
state-approved programs, 87
teaching profession and, 75
training schools for nurses, 15 ff.
unemployment and, 70
women's development of, 12-13, 35-36
in World War II, 45
Education Committee of NLNE, 44
Elementary education, 71
Environment
    community, 210-12, 226 ff.
    family, 140-42, 153
    pesticides and, 67
    technology and, 67, 68, 210
Episodic career patterns, 274
Equal Suffrage Act, 37
Ethnic groups, 138, 150
European immigrants, 33
Evaluation of
    alternative choices for reaching goals,
        242 ff.
    community nursing plan, 261 ff.
    education, 46-47, 53, 79, 82-83
    family care plan, 188 ff.
    focus and emphasis, 264
    goals, 189-91, 262-63
    nursing needs, 262-63
    observable behavior, 263
    total plan, 189
Examinations for licensure, 84
Experimentation, educational, 274

Facilities, community, 151, 221, 231, 232,
        233
    availability, 179-80, 183-84, 221, 233,
        234
    coordination of, 185-87, 257
    data on, 214-15
    duplication of services, 214
    existing, 215 ff., 251, 258, 260
    goals and, 167
    mobilization of, 256-57
    personnel, 231
    planning groups and, 214-15
    referrals and, 183-84
Family, 117 ff.
    age and, 133
    assigned roles, 167
    basic assumptions about, 160-61
    as basic unit of society, 119-20
    budgeting, 168
    characteristics, 132 ff.
    conceptual frameworks for, 146-47
    contacts with nurse, 174, 180

Family (cont.)
    cultural factors, 137-38, 179
    daily activities, 134-36
    data, 130 ff.
        base line of, 130-31, 149, 154, 162-
            63, 177-78
    decision-making, 134-35, 149-50, 172
    defining health problems, 148-49, 153
    definition of, 119
    dependency and independence of, 168,
        173
    developmental stage of, 132, 147
    dynamics, 121-22
    eating patterns, 135-36, 171
    economic status, 137-38, 150, 167, 168
    education, 150
    environment, 140-42, 153
    ethnic group, 138, 150
    evaluation of care plan for, 188 ff.
    federal legislation and, 125-26
    financial costs of nursing, 167
    functions, definition of, 119
    goals, 159-60, 165, 166 ff.
        evaluation of, 189-91
        health maintenance and promotion,
            169-71
        reality of, 190
    health nurse, future for, 273
    help sources, 143, 178
    housing, 140-41, 153
    identification of nursing needs, 152-54
    implementation of plan for, 176 ff.
    income, 137-38, 150
    individual health relationship to, 160
    institutional approach to, 140, 147
    interaction approach, 146-47
    interrelatedness of health problems, 155
    knowledge about health, 150, 164-65
    larger community and, 180
    leisure time, 136-37
    medical history, 154
    model, 162
    multiple needs of, 163-64
    neighborhood, 141, 167, 182
    nuclear, 120-21, 168, 173
    nurse's view vs. family view, 166
    parental roles, 133-34
    patterns, shaping and molding forces,
        120
    planning care for, 159 ff.
    position in time, 133
    priority of nursing needs, 164-66
    provision of services for, 180-81
    public health movement and, 51
    reading for information, 165
    referrals and collaboration for care of,
        183-84
    relatives, 182

Family (cont.)
    religion, 138-39, 150
    roles and relationships, 133, 149, 167
    sex, 133
    significant others, 140, 178
    situational approach to, 147
    size, 133
    sleeping patterns, 135
    solution of problems, 156
    source for medical care, 167-68
    specialization and, 122-23
    strengths and weaknesses, 164
    structure-function approach, 147
    threat-avoiding needs, 165
    transportation, 141, 180
    as unit of service, 54, 117, 119-20, 186
    value system, 139-40, 151, 179
Father, decision-making and, 134
Federal government
    civil rights and, 77
    community and, 95, 199, 208, 223, 243
    comprehensive health centers and, 113
    educational funds, 72-73, 112
    family as patient and, 125-26
    national health plan and, 110
    New Deal and, 62
    poverty program, 107
    public health and, 49, 53
    railroad assistance, 8
    regionalization and, 245
    relief projects, 89
    social legislation, 76 ff.
    transportation and, 65
    welfare and, 76
Federal Highways Act (1921), 31
Federation of Women's Clubs, 14
Finances. See Economics; Federal govern-
        ment; Funds.
Flapper era, 37
Flexner Study, 35
Fluoridation, 211
Focus of community health nursing, 162,
        264, 271
Fogarty, John, 123
Food habits, 135-36, 171
Ford, Henry, 30, 32
Foundations, 38-39
Frances Payne Bolton School of Nursing, 46
Funds. See also Federal government.
    agency, 217, 242-43
    Cadet Corps, 80
    community, 39, 76, 223
    educational, 52, 73
    public health, first census of, 54-55
    relief project, 89
    social consciousness and, 76
    Social Security Act and, 89-90
Future of community health nursing, 269 ff.

Garbage disposal, 211, 228
Gardner, John, 198
Gardner, Mary, 43
"Generalized specialist," 185, 272
Geographic location, 222
Germ theory, 48-49
Ghetto areas, 106, 210
G.I. Bill, 72, 81
Goals
   budgeting, 168
   community, 240 ff., 262-63
   comprehensive care, 241
   educational, 84
   evaluation of, 189-91, 242 ff., 262
   family, 159-60, 165, 166 ff., 189-91
   key factors, 246
   priority of, 170
   reality of, 190
   revising plan and, 182
   short-term, 170-71, 247 ff.
   unanticipated outcomes and, 190
Goldmark, Josephine, 46
Goods, production and distribution of,
     30, 66, 67
Government
   community, 208
   federal. See Federal government.
Grading of nursing schools, 46-47, 53
Graduate programs, 47, 112
   development of, 35
   enrollment, 88
   federal support, 73
   first, 13
   specialization and, 95
Great Society, 77-78, 198
Greenbie, M. B., 5
Group, planning, 240
Guatemala, 67
Guidance, 258

Hampton, Isabel, 17
"Handmaiden of physician" image, 97
Hanlon, J., 217
Harnish, T., 249
Health
   care system
     availability of, 179-80, 221, 233, 234
     change in, 200, 260-61
     coordination of, 185-87, 219, 221,
       257, 259
     criteria for, 221-22
     delivery system, 260-61, 269-70
     demands on, 81, 203, 270-71
     development of better, 199
     federal funds for, 89-90
     personnel, 256
   definition of, 118

Health (cont.)
   departments
     community, 92, 254-55
     future of, 113
     organizational patterns, 92
     role of, 94-95
     state, 89-90
   facilities, community, 151, 178-80
     See also Facilities, community.
   insurance, national, 91
   maintenance and promotion goals, 169-
     71
   problems
     data on, 130 ff., 230 ff. See also
      Data.
     delineation of, 148, 153
     history of family, 142-44
     individual, 155
     patterns of, 165-66, 213
     public health role in, 94-95
   professionals. See Professionals.
   workers
     changing role of, 118
     demand for, 81
     duplication of functions, 177
     roles and relationships, 177
     specialization, 122-23, 272-73
     teams, 110, 177
Help sources for family, 143, 178
Henry Street Settlement, 21, 50
Higher education. See also Colleges and
     universities.
   development of, 12-13, 34-36
   first Department of Nursing and Health,
     52
   nursing programs, 42-43, 47, 84-86
High schools
   college preparation and, 71
   1900 to New Deal, 34
Highways, 64
Hilleboe, H. E., 199
Historical background
   from 1865 to 1900, 3 ff.
   from 1900 to New Deal, 29 ff.
   New Deal through Johnson era, 62 ff.
History
   community, 208, 223-24
   family medical, 142-44, 154
Home care programs, 91, 179, 255
Home economics, 35-36
Home health agency, certified, 215-16
Hoover, Herbert, 31, 41
Hospital Survey and Construction Act
     (1946), 91
Hospitals
   citizens groups and, 24-25
   Civil War and, 6
   extension of services, 255, 258

Hospitals (cont.)
    as focus of nursing, 58-59
    training of nurses, 15 ff., 48
Housing
    community and, 210-11, 227
    family and, 140-41, 153
Humanitarianism, 24, 57
Husband, decision-making and, 134

Idealism, 24, 57
Identification of nursing needs
    for community, 220 ff.
    for family, 152-54
Illness patterns of community, 213
Immigration
    from 1865 to 1900, 10-11
    from 1900 to New Deal, 33
    after 1930, 69
    limitation of, 33
Implementation of plan, 176 ff., 251 ff.
    ascertaining resources and, 254-56
    base-line data and, 253
    change and, 252
    for community, 251 ff.
    decisions about, 178-80
    evaluation of, 188 ff., 261
    for family, 150-51, 176 ff.
    overlapping with planning, 176-77
    personnel and, 256
    revising plan and, 181-83
Income
    community and, 226
    family, 137-38, 150
Independence of family, 168, 173
Individual
    economic security of community re-
        lated to, 53
    as focus of service, 117-18
    health problems, 155, 160
    medical model and, 125
    in nuclear family, 121
    public health movement and, 50
Individualism, education and, 13
Industrialization
    from 1865 to 1900, 9
    from 1900 to New Deal, 31-33
    New Deal to Johnson era, 65 ff.
    in 1970s, 107
Infant
    mortality, 109, 230
    welfare stations, 50
Information. See Data.
Initiative, 173, 238
Institutional approach to family, 147
Institutional nursing, as focus, 59-60
Instructive District Nursing, coinage of title,
    19

Instructive District Nursing Association, 19,
    52
Insulin, 172-73
Insurance, compulsory national health, 91
Interaction approach, 146-47
Interagency referrals, 248-49, 259
Interstate Commerce Act, 8

Jacques, M., 18
Jenkins, Helen, 52
Job description of agency director, 217
John Hancock Life Insurance Company, 91
Johns Hopkins University, 13
Johnson, L. B., 77-78
Junior colleges, 71
    first, 34

Kellogg Foundation, 88
Kennedy, J. F., 77
Key factors for nursing needs, 246
Key people, communications and, 212, 229,
    263
King, Larry L., 77
King, Martin Luther, Jr., 77
Klein, D., 195, 196
Knowledge explosion, 111, 185
    specialization and, 272

Labor force
    depression and, 40
    from 1865 to 1900, 10
    strikes, 66
    unionization, 32, 65-66
    women in, 37, 74, 108
Ladies Aid Societies, 5, 15
Lay people, working with, 161
Leadership, 128, 238
Lee, C. B. T., 78
Legislation, 95
    civil rights, 77
    community and, 199, 223
    education and, 42
    family as patient and, 125-26
    national health plan and, 110
    poverty programs, 78, 107
    regionalization and, 245
    social, 76 ff.
Leisure time, 136-37
Lent, Mary, 45
Licensure, 83-84
Life expectancy
    in Civil War, 6
    in 1900, 33
    women's, 74
    in World War II, 90

Location of community, 222
Long-term goals, 247 ff.
Los Angeles settlement, 22
Lysaught Report, 112

Manpower needs, 126-27, 218
Marriage, necessity of, 108
Mass distribution of goods, 67
Mass production, 30, 66
Master's programs, 84, 87, 88, 112
Maternal health program, 241
McIver, Pearl, 89
Meal patterns, 135-36, 171
Media, 212, 227
Medical care. *See also* Health care system.
    for family, 167-68
    knowledge explosion and, 111
    in 1970s, 109
Medical education, early, 16
Medical history of family, 142-44, 154
Medical model
    family care plan, 162
    nursing and, 124-25
Medical technology, 68-69
Medicare, 110, 215, 243, 252
Men, nursing education standards and, 58
Methylmercury, 67
Metropolitan Life Insurance Company, 51, 91
Military
    technology and, 68
    •women in, 74, 80
Mobility, 69, 223
Mobilization of resources, 256-57
Model
    cities, 107, 261
    family, 162
    medical, nursing and, 124-25
    for organization, 92
Model-T, 30
Monopolies, 31-32
Montag, Mildred, 82
Montefiore Home Care Program, 91
Morrill Act (1944), 72
Mother
    decision-making and, 134
    nursing care by, 173-74
Movies, 32-33
Mowry, G., 74
Multidisciplinary health care, 177, 253

National Commission on Community Services, 221, 244
National Commission for the Study of Nursing and Nursing Education, 88, 112, 274
National Council for War Services, 82

National Defense Education Act, 73
National Education Association, 79
National Emergency Committee on Nursing, 44
National health insurance, 91
National health plan, 110
National League for Nursing
    accreditation
        of community health nursing services, 95, 113, 216
        of education programs, 83
    college programs support, 86
    formation of, 82
National League for Nursing Education, 47, 82
    examinations for licensure, 84
    founding of, 44
    World War II and, 80
National Mental Health Act, 85
National Nursing Accreditation Service, 83
National Nursing Council, 80, 81-82
National Organization for Public Health Nursing, 55
    census, first, 54, 55
    educational standards, 52-53, 83
    foundation of, 43-44
    World War II and, 80
National Origins Act (1924), 33
National Student Nurse Association, 82
National Youth Administration, 70, 72
Navy Nurse Corps, 80
Needs, nursing. *See* Nursing needs.
Negro education, 71, 73
Neighborhood, 141, 150, 167, 182
    health center staff, 260
New Frontier, 77
New Haven Hospital, 15
New York City
    first school nurse in, 50
    health department, 41
    Puerto Rican immigration, 69
    visiting nurse services, 91
New York State licensure, 83
Nightingale, Florence, 7, 14, 15
Noise, 229
North Carolina, 42
Nuclear family, 120-21
    dependency of, 168, 173
Nurses
    community health, 114. *See also* Community health nurse.
    employed in public health, 127
    family health, future for, 273
    legislative influence of, 42
    role in 1970s, 111
    unemployment, 79
Nurses' Associated Alumnae Association, 17, 43

Nursing
    action. *See* Action, nursing.
    care, by mother, 173-74
    care system. *See* Health care system;
        Plan, nursing care.
    conceptual frameworks, 146-47, 221
    diagnosis, definition of, 152
    educational programs, 87. *See also*
        Colleges and universities; Educa-
        tion.
    historical development
        from 1865 to 1900, 14 ff.
        from 1900 to New Deal, 41 ff.
        New Deal to Johnson era, 79 ff.
    licensure, 83-84
    medical model, 124-25
    needs
        availability of services and, 234
        definition of, 152
        evaluation of, 262
        as focus, 160, 162
        goals and, 168. *See also* Goals.
        identification of, 152-54, 220 ff.
        key factors for, 246
        other needs, relationship to, 163-64
        preplanning and, 239-40
        priority of, 164-66, 234
        statement of, 156-57
    organizations, leadership responsibility,
        43
    practical, 84, 87
    priorities, 112-13
    process, interrelatedness of steps in,
        152, 176-77, 182
    prognosis, definition of, 152
    psychiatric, 85
    research, 60, 85, 87, 111, 147
        future for, 275-76
Nursing Council of National Defense, 80
Nursing Research, 85
Nutting, Adelaide, 42, 44
Nyquist, Ewald B., 68

Observable behavior, 263
Office of Economic Opportunity, 78
Official agencies, 254-55
Organizational patterns, 92
Organized community effort, 197, 202
Oshkosh, Wisconsin, 196
Outcomes. *See also* Goals.
    evaluation of, 189-91, 263
Overcrowding, 227
Overlapping of resources, 94, 176-77, 214

Parents
    decision-making and, 134-35
    missing, 134
    roles, 133-34

Peace Corps, 77, 109
People, information about, 209-10
Perception of family health problems, 165-
        66
Personnel, community health, 217-18, 231
    data analysis and, 233-34
    implementation of plan and, 256
    neighborhood health center, 260
    utilization of, 218
Pesticides, 67
Philadelphia, 20
Philanthropy, 11, 13
Physicians
    educational standards and, 58
    settlements and, 21
    women, early, 15
Plan, nursing care
    for community, 236 ff.
        activating, 257 ff.
        alternatives, 247, 248-49
        comprehensive care and, 241
        coordination of, 259
        decision-making, 199-200, 239
        definition of, 237
        development of, 236 ff.
        evaluation of, 261 ff.
        existing services and, 215 ff., 251,
            258, 260
        expanding programs and, 258
        facilities and, 214-15
        federal government and, 199
        goals, key factors for, 246
        guidelines for, 237-38
        implementation of, 251 ff.
        initiative in, 238
        kind and number of planners, 239-
            40
        politics and, 243
        preplanning and, 199, 239-40
        regionalization and, 245
        as social action, 237
        steps for, 238-39, 246 ff.
        timing for, 244
        totality of information and, 245
        unanticipated problems, 252-53
        urgency of, 237
        vested interests and, 243
    for family, 159 ff.
        availability of facilities and, 167-68
        base-line information, 162-63, 177-
            78
        collaboration, 162, 183-84
        decision-making, 160-61, 178-80
        development of, 148 ff., 159 ff.
        evaluation of, 188 ff.
        goals, 159-60, 166 ff.
        implementation of, 148, 150-51,
            176 ff.
        medical model, 162
        multiple needs and, 163-64

Plan, nursing care (cont.)
  for family (cont.)
    overlapping, 176-77
    priority of needs and, 164-66
    referrals and, 183-84
    revision of, 181-83
    source of medical care and, 167-68
    values of family and, 179
Policies, agency, 123-24, 127
Politics, 243
Pollution, technology and, 68
Population
  characteristics of community, 208, 209,
    224-26
  distribution, 224-25
  in 1860, 4
  from 1865 to 1900, 11
  from 1900 to New Deal, 33
  New Deal to Johnson era, 69-70
  in 1970s, 105
Position Paper on Education for Nursing,
    85-86
Postgraduate programs, 47-48, 53, 88
Poverty, 201, 202, 210
  district nursing development and, 18 ff.
  programs, 78, 107, 243
  urbanization and, 70
Practical nursing, 84, 87
Pregnancy, 246, 258
Preplanning
  decision-making and, 199-200
  nursing needs and, 239-40
Press, 212
Prevention of disease, 169-71, 214
Priorities, 112-13
  nursing needs and, 164-66, 170, 234
Production of goods, 30, 66
Professionalism, progress toward, 99
Professionals
  consumer demands on, 161
  continuing development of, 187
  educational programs and, 73, 84
  family perception of, 144
  role of others, 181
  women, 75
Profile, community, 208
Prognosis, nursing, definition of, 152
Prohibition, 36
Protective programs, 202
Protective services, 211, 228
Psychiatric nursing, 85
Public education, 12, 34
Public health
  change of goals in, 201
  definitions of, 201-202
  nurses employed in, 127
Public health nursing
  accreditation of educational programs
    in, 93
  availability of, 126

census, first, 54-55
cost studies, first, 55
defensive role of, 93
definition of, 95, 114
  by ANA, 93-94
  first use of term, 21
Depression and, 55
duplication of responsibilities, 94
family as unit of service and, 186
future for, 113
goals, 242
historical development
  from 1865 to 1900, 18 ff.
  from 1900 to New Deal, 48 ff.
  New Deal to Johnson era, 88 ff.
manual, first, 55
organizational patterns, 92
postgraduate courses, 53
qualifications established, 55
ratio of nurses, 92
relief projects, 89
Public Health Service
  consultation services, 89
  World War II and, 80
Puerto Rican immigration, 69

Radio, 32
Railroads, 8
Rathbone, William, 20
Reading, information from, 165
Recruitment, nursing, 43, 44
Red Cross, 45
Referrals, 183-84, 249-50, 259
Reform movement, 37-39
  educational, 12
  labor, 32
  public health, 49-50
  zenith of, 58
Regional Medical Programs Act, 199, 245
Regionalization, 110, 245
Registered nurse
  educational programs, 87
  licensure, 84
  number of (in 1968), 110
Rehabilitation, 183
Relatives, 143, 182
Relief agencies, 41, 89
Religion, 138-39, 150
Reorganization of established services, 260
Research, nursing, 85, 87, 111
  beginnings of, 60
  conceptual frameworks, 147
  educational, 276
  future for, 275-76
Resources, community, 231. See also
    Facilities, community.
  ascertaining, 254-56
  availability, 179-80, 183-84, 221, 233,
    234

Resources, community (cont.)
    data on, 214-15
    existing, 215 ff., 251, 258, 260
    expansion of, 258
    mobilization of, 256-57
    nursing needs and, 234
    referrals and, 183-84
Revising care plan, 181-83
Richards, Linda, 15
Robb, Isabel Hampton, 17
Roberts, M. M., 17
Robischon, P., 203
Rockefeller Foundation, 35, 39, 46
Rockefeller, Nelson, 68
Roles
    family, 133, 149, 167
    health workers, 177
Roosevelt, Theodore, 37
Rosenwald Foundation, 39
Rudd, Robert, 67
Rural waste disposal, 211

Sanders, I. T., 195
Sanitary Commission, 5
Sanitation, 211, 228
Satellite clinics, 255, 258
Scholarships, 72
School nurse, first, 50
Schools of nursing. See also Colleges and
        universities; Education.
    central, 81
    college and university relationship, 42-
        43, 47, 84-86
    grading of, 46-47
    graduate, first, 13
    historical development, 15 ff.
        in 1893, 17
        early 1900s, 42
        in 1920s, 46-47
        in World War II, 45
    legislation and, 42
    recruitment, 43
Secondary education, 34, 71
Segregation, 71
Servicemen's Readjustment Act, 72
Services, nursing
    provision of, for family, 180-81
    variety of, in community, 254
Settlements, 20 ff., 38
Sewage disposal, 211, 228
Sex characteristics, 133, 209
Shaw, Anna Howard, 45
Shelter, 140-41
Shephard-Towner Act (1924), 53
Short-term goals, 170-71, 247 ff.
Side effects of implementation, 190
Significant others, 140, 143, 178

Silent Spring, 67-68
Simmons College, 52
Situational approach to family, 147
Sleeping patterns, 135
Slums
    from 1865 to 1900, 10-11
    settlement houses, 20 ff., 38
Smith-Lever Act (1914), 35
Social action, 237
Social consciousness, 37-39, 75
Social legislation, 76 ff.
Social revolution in 1970s, 108
Social Security Act (1935), 89-90
Social system, community as, 194-95
Social unit, nuclear family as, 119 ff.
Societal contacts of family, 140
Society, manpower needs of, 126-27
Society of Superintendents of Training
        Schools for Nurses, 17, 44, 52
Socioeconomic status of family, 137-38,
        150
Sources of help for family, 167-68, 178
Southern Regional Education Board, 84
Specialization
    communicable diseases and, 49-50
    coordinating services and, 185
    family and, 122-23
    future for, 275-76
    "generalized," 185, 272
    graduate programs, 95
    knowledge explosion and, 272
    need for, 86
Staff. See Personnel, community health.
Standard Curriculum for Nursing Schools,
        44
Standards, educational, 52-53
State
    -approved nursing education programs,
        87
    consultation services, 89
    health departments, funds for, 89-90
    licensing laws, 83-84
State Board Test Pool, 84
State Charities Aid Association of New
        York, 15
Statistical problems in first census of public
        health nurses, 55
Status
    automobile and, 30
    socioeconomic, 137-38, 150
    women's. See Women, status of.
Stereotypes, decision-making, 134-35
Stewart, Isabel, 44
Stock market crash, 40
Strikes, labor, 66
Structure-function approach, 147
Student
    federal assistance to, 72

Student (cont.)
   nursing care, 79
   unrest, 73, 78
Subcommittee on Hospitals, 45
Suburbanization, 70, 106
Suffrage, women's, 36-37
Supervisors, qualifications for, 55, 217
Supreme Court decisions
   industry and, 32
   separate but equal education, 71
   workers and, 32
Surgeon General, 49
Sweden, 67, 109

Taft-Hartley Act (1947), 66
Taylor, Carl, 195
Teachers, 75
   future for, 275
Teachers College, Columbia University,
   43, 52
Team, health, 110, 177
Technology
   communications, 229
   continuing professional development
      and, 187
   environment and, 67, 68, 210
   historical development
      from 1865 to 1900, 9
      from 1900 to New Deal, 31-33, 35
      New Deal to Johnson era, 65 ff.
      in 1970s, 106-107
   medical, 68-69
   military, 68
   working women and, 13-14
Television, 66-67, 212-13
Threat-avoiding needs, 165
Time, family position in, 133
Timing in community planning, 244
Title VI of Social Security Act, 89-90
Totality of information, 245
Training schools for nurses. *See also* Col-
      leges and universities; Education.
   early, 15 ff.
   federal funds for, 90
   university, beginnings of, 42-43
Transportation
   community, 212, 228-29
   family and, 141, 181
   historical development
      from 1865 to 1900, 8-9
      from 1900 to New Deal, 30-31
      New Deal to Johnson era, 64-65
   noise, 229
Trash disposal, 211, 228
Trusts, 31-32
Tuberculosis, 49-50
Typhoid fever, 49

Unanticipated problems
   evaluation of goals and, 190
   in plan of action, 252-53
Unemployment
   depression and, 40, 48
   education and, 70
   in 1970s, 107
   nursing, 79
   women and, 74
Unionization, 32, 65-66
Unit of service, family as, 54, 117, 119-20,
   186
United Funds, 242
United States Public Health Service, 80, 89
United States Sanitary Commission, 5
University. *See also* Colleges and univer-
      sities.
   beginnings of training in, 42-43, 47
   curricula, 35
   first Department of Nursing and Health,
      52
Urbanization. *See also* Cities.
   transportation and, 64
   waste disposal, 211

Value system, 139-140, 151, 179
Vassar College, 6
Vassar Training Camp, 45
Vested interests, 243
Vickers, J., 165
Vietnam war, 73, 78
Visiting nurse associations
   beginnings of, 20 ff., 59-60
   change and, 259-60
   college and university collaboration
      with, 52
   future of, 113
   implementation of plan and, 254
   insurance and, 91
   public health movement and, 51
Visiting Nurse Society of Philadelphia, 20
Visits, nursing, 174, 180, 184
Vital statistics, 213, 230
Vocational nursing programs, 87
Volstead Act (1920), 36
Voluntary health agencies
   communicable diseases and, 49
   development of, 19 ff., 39, 59-60, 89
   goals for, 242
   national, 76-77
   as resource, 254
Volunteers in Service to America (VISTA),
      77, 107, 109

Wages, Ford and, 32
Wald, Lillian, 21, 50, 51

Waste disposal, 211, 228
Water supply, 211, 228
Welfare programs, 50, 76, 78
Western Regional Board of Higher Education, 84
Western Reserve University, 46, 52
West Pakistan, 67
Wife, decision-making and, 134
Wilson, Woodrow, 37, 44
Winch, R. F., 119
Winslow, C.-E. A., 46, 50, 201
Women
    in armed forces, 74
    colleges, development of, 12-13, 35-36
    equality struggle, 36-37, 74
    life expectancy, 74
    physicians, early, 15
    professional, 75
    status of
        Civil War and, 4 ff.

Women (cont.)
    from 1865 to 1900, 13-14
    from 1900 to New Deal, 36-37
    New Deal to Johnson era, 74-75
    unemployment and, 74
    working, 13, 74, 108
Women's Committee of National Defense, 37
Women's Education Association, 19-20
Workers. See Health workers; Labor force.
Working conditions, early, 10-11, 79
World Health Organization, 91
World War I, 37, 44-45
World War II, 80, 90, 96

Yale University School of Nursing, 46

Zakrzewska, Marie, 15

DATE DUE

SEP 26 '77		
NOV 28 '77		
JUN 27 '79		
FEB 25 '82		
FEB 11 1983		
FEB. 20. 1984		
FEB 9 1987		
JUL 4 1996		